Vitamins and You
You

Hair, Skin and Nails

Disclaimer

What will you find in this book?

The *Vitamins and You: Beauty* Book contains the following:

1. Clear and descriptive vitamin recipes for beauty.
2. Accurate information on the benefits of each type of vitamin.
3. Benefits of vitamins for different age groups i.e. teens and older women.

Table of Contents

Contents

The Lead in - Vitamins

Vitamins are basically chemicals that make up a big part of our body's processes. They are a vital component in the reactions that take part inside our cells. Each type is responsible for performing a specific function in the body.

It is important to know what supplements your body needs and make sure that you have an adequate intake of them. This is particularly important for essential nutrients which our bodies may need extra help in getting. For example, our bodies cannot make Vitamin D and that is why its needs its quota from the foods you eat, the supplements that you take or regular exposure to the sunlight.

Moreover at certain stages in your life you will need specific vitamins in different quantities. As we age, the needs of our body continually changes especially in terms of vitamins and minerals. When you cannot get enough of a particular one that you need you may incur some serious illnesses.

Although many of us have heard and read and promised ourselves that we would follow the 5 servings of fruit and vegetables each day practice, we don't because it is simply not that easy. We have our jobs, the family and that leaves little time for ourselves. This is especially true for women; with the family and sometimes even jobs to take care of, many do not find the time to maintain their own health.

When we say vitamins are a huge deal- we do mean huge. Without vitamins we would not be able to breathe, think, digest food or walk our dog. Given our hectic lifestyles chances are that you are not getting enough of the good stuff. Sometimes, we simply don't have the time to prepare a nutritious meal of even have the time to eat our recommended servings of fruits and vegetables.

Many companies often claim that their products can give you amazing results with the benefits of all the vitamins in one but it will be in your best interests to ignore them. You see, most nutritional supplements and 'cosmeceuticals' – a fusion of the word cosmetics and pharmaceutical's intended for makeup with added medicinal benefits - are tested for safety mainly and not for the benefits they yield. This means that a product can effectively be useless, and not be taken off the shelves as long as it isn't doing any harm. This is why looking at independent studies or researching a particular brand is important.

Even though a product's package may say that it comes with its own share of useful antioxidants and other nutrients sometimes the packaging and labeling may be obscure as to how much of a certain ingredient there might be in it. This book will show you how to make the best out of your diet and supplements and reveal that not all of them are created equal.

What Types of Vitamins are there?

Vitamins are organic compounds which the body cannot make on its own, therefore we need to get them from external sources such as diet or sunlight exposure.

While it may seem that most of the vitamins have been discovered yet there are still some scientists out there who think that there may be more undiscovered vitamins. Health in general is a forever changing field of science and with new technologies that arise; more discoveries are constantly being made.

At present there are only less than 20 recognized vitamins which are broken into two categories: fat soluble and water-soluble.

Water-soluble vitamins do not store in the body for very long and are expelled in our urine. Vitamins B and C are water-soluble. These are replaced extremely easily and need to be replenished in our diet daily in order to have their maximum efficacy in our body.

Fat-soluble vitamins can be stored in the fat reserves of our body. These can stay in the body for days, weeks or months. These are usually the ones which you can overdose on if you are not careful. These are A D, E and K.

A Brief History of Vitamins

Vitamins were first introduced into the scientific community in 1912 by Casimir Funk who originally described them as 'vitamines,' however knowledge of their presence was well known before that. In fact, many significant discoveries about vitamins were made in the early nineteenth century.

While each vitamin was discovered by different groups of chemists, physiologists, physicians and epidemiologists, there have all been driven by their common interest in health and disease.

These discoveries arose from the fundamental need to discover the reason behind the difference in nutritional value of certain foods in animal studies. At the time many scientists were merely looking at food as a source of carbohydrates, proteins and fats. It was then discovered at the turn of the 20th century, that other organic compounds found in foods were vital for maintaining normal nutrition and had to be more carefully explored.

It so followed that there was an urgent demand to discover these organic substances which were very specific in nature. They were found to have specific functions away from the normal energy sources of carbohydrates, protein and fats.

There were many events in history which pointed to the value of vitamins, these included diaries from the 18th century of explorers suffering from scurvy, or adventurers suffering from malnutrition when placed on certain staples for months on end. Despite this, the first noted experiments of vitamins are generally regarded to have been performed by Nikolai Lunin in 1881 who only fed mice protein, carbohydrate and fats. After the mice failed to survive he recorded that something as natural as milk would need to have other substances in it essential to life.

However, instead of seeking what these compounds were, Lunin's superiors believed that the protein extracted from the milk was of a poorer quality. It wasn't until 14 years later that Cornelius Pekelharing revisited the experiments and came to the conclusion that there was more to milk and other foods than just merely carbohydrates, protein and fats.

Christian Eijkman and Sir Frederick Hopkins then went on to examine the subject of vitamins and the resulting diseases that arose from their deficiency. Their combined efforts over decades of assimilating information and researching culminated in being the co-recipients of the Nobel Prize for Medicine in 1929.

In 1937 Paul Karrer in his Nobel Prize lecture for chemistry further investigated what this new substance actually did in the body. He stated that even though scientists had doubted the material specificity of vitamins and what they actually were, there was no doubt that they played an important role in nutrition and maintaining the integrity of many chemical processes in the body.

Important Vitamins for Beauty

Vitamin A

Vitamin A was probably named after the first alphabet for being an overachiever. It' s an antioxidant that corrects vision, lowers the risk of cardiac disease and is known as the fountain of youth as studies have shown that substantial amounts can make your skin look substantially younger. It is known as the 'gold standard' when it comes to treating wrinkles, fine lines, taking away the roughness from your skin and age spots.

Vitamin A is considered a very important anti-oxidant vitamin. Use of Vitamin A in the form of Beta-carotene kills free radicals and keeps you looking more youthful. Vitamin A is used regularly for the treatment of acne.

Topical Vitamin A derivatives dry the skin and peel the upper layers off. This quality is very useful in treating acne as it helps to reduce the amount of sebum that stays on the face for prolonged periods of time. Sebum, the skin oil is the most responsible for causing acne. This sebum becomes infected and forms acne. Vitamin A derivatives dry out this sebum on the site of application and prevent it from blocking the pores. The other main cause of acne formation is blocked sebaceous glands. Once the top layer begins peeling due to the effects of Vitamin A derivatives, the pores open making the formation of acne pustules difficult.

The side-effects of Vitamin A are very dangerous, especially when they are used during pregnancy. For those who are pregnant or are planning to get pregnant should consult their doctor before using any Vitamin A derivative or Vitamin A itself as it is a known teratogen if taken in excess. Teratogens are responsible for causing major birth defects.

In products Vitamin A is known by any of the following and can be found in a wide range of foods, hair care or skincare:

- Retinol
- Retinal
- Retinoic Acid
- Retinyl esters
- Tretinoin
- Adapalene
- Tazarotene

Other benefits of Vitamin A include the maintenance of cells in the body, which studies have shown can possibly help with the reduction of cancer, it can prove useful in the treatment of measles and can prevent you from having issues with your eyes in the later stages of your life.

DAILY RECOMMENDED DOSE (general): 2300 IU (international units) please make sure you look at the Federal Drugs and Administration (FDA) guidelines to make sure of the dosage you should be taking.

Thinking you may require supplementation does not mean that you can hit your nearest drugstore and start and clear out the Vitamin A supplement aisle. It can prove toxic if taken in large doses. A toxic amount of Vitamin A in the body is known as Hypervitaminosis A and can lead to symptoms such as dizziness, nausea and indigestion right through to more severe manifestations such as cirrhosis (scarring of the liver) or bleeding lungs. The symptoms are wide and varied even though Vitamin A toxicity is quite rare.

A deficiency in Vitamin A, while also rare, can lead to problems such as a decrease in the ability to see at night time, age-related macular degeneration or a decrease in the ability to see in general.

Usually you won't have to worry about a deficiency if you are getting enough from fortified foods such as fortified milk or having regular serves of fruit and vegetables. Supplements should always be taken with caution and you need to make a note of what you are taking so that you can inform your doctor if there are any interactions.

Vitamin A is important for your beauty due to the fact that it helps with the constant renewal of skin cells. This means that the old cells can slough off easier giving way to newer, younger looking cells. This is why Vitamin A is a regular additive in many skincare products.

The best sources of Vitamin A are beta carotene sources like cantaloupe, carrots, liver and fish oils. Other sources include leafy green vegetables, orange and yellow vegetables, broccoli and squash.

Tips when using Vitamin A

Be careful when using prescription bought Vitamin A derivatives as they are far harsher than what you will find in over the counter medication. Usually prescription Vitamin A products will accelerate the rate in which you see result – about 1 to 2 months. However, they may cause redness, itchiness and irritation when used topically in dosages which are too high for the sensitivity of your skin.

Over the counter Vitamin A treatments are best for those who are just starting to apply Vitamin A to their face. You can gradually build up to using products which contain more as your body grows accustomed to it.

Not everyone's skin is the same therefore make sure you always test the product you are about to buy on the inside of your wrist first to see if there is a reaction before you apply it to your face. Your skin will gradually adjust to using Vitamin A but initially you may experience some discomfort. When using it topically, use small amounts to test how your skin will react to it. If there is too much redness or irritation either use a smaller dose or discontinue use.

Most retinol treatments will suggest that you avoid exposure to sunlight while using the product as the efficiency of topical Vitamin A products reduces greatly with exposure to the sunlight. This is why it is recommended that you use these products before you sleep at night. This is why Vitamin A is commonly found in skin creams and your night rejuvenation formulas.

Vitamin B

There are eight B vitamins in total and they are responsible for maintaining your muscle tone and metabolism and keeping your mind sharp. For women the Vitamin B subtype that should make their top priority list is Folic Acid which keeps red blood cells healthy and shields the body against any possible birth defects and cancer.

Because there are so many different Vitamin B complexes it is quite a complex vitamin to cover. This will be discussed in a different section however the basics will be covered here.

Vitamin B is known as the following in it different forms:

- Thiamine (B1)
- Riboflavin
- Niacin
- Pantothenic acid
- Biotin
- Vitamin B6 (pyridoxine)
- Folate (called folic acid when included in supplements)
- Vitamin B12 (cyanocobalamin)

These are the eight different types of Vitamin B and they are crucial in the production of energy for the body, blood cells and maintaining healthy brain function. Taking Vitamin B supplements while pregnant can also help to prevent Spina bifida in infants.

A deficiency in Vitamin B can lead to anemia and its related symptoms such as fatigue, breathlessness, frequent headaches and irritability. A lack of Vitamin B12 has been linked to mild forms of depression or lack of concentration as it is important for the productions of neurotransmitters in the brain needed for the regulation of mood and memory.

Too much Vitamin B, especially B6 can result in nerve damage. Too much B12 can cause diahorrea, itching, blood clots and allergic reactions however this is uncommon unless you are take specific injections of these supplements.

DAILY FOLATE DOSE: 400 mcg (up to 600mcg if you are pregnant).

You do not necessarily need supplements of Vitamin B if you are not pregnant or planning to be. This is because B vitamins can be commonly found in fortified foods or from a balanced diet. You can find them in grains, breakfast cereals, beans, asparagus and whole grain breads.

The B Vitamins are important for cells throughout your body. This includes the skin cells as well. It is important that you get foods that are rich in this like fortified grain products, eggs and chicken. Without sufficient B Vitamins you will be faced with dry and itchy skin.

Tips when using Vitamin B

Vitamin B3 (niacinamide) should be used in the morning and the evening. It is useful in helping with the irritation caused by Vitamin A topical products. You can mix the two together to help reduce any irritation that may occur and boost their effectiveness at the same time.

Vitamin C

Most of you know it as a remedy for the common cold. But did you know that this particular vitamin has never proven to cure or prevent this common ailment? However, this antioxidant works to improve your immune system which in turn helps prevent heart diseases, prenatal problems and eye issues. It accelerates your ability to heal and does what Botox fails at: naturally fending off wrinkles.

A shortage in Vitamin C has been historically known to cause scurvy, a condition that can cause the loss of your teeth, haemorrhage, bruising, weakening of inability to fight infection, mild anemia, and bleeding. An essential amount of Vitamin C is necessary to promote overall health and wellbeing. In many instances a nutritious and well-balanced diet may be enough, but when it is not, vitamin supplementation necessary to take care of the deficiency.

Vitamin C is constantly marketed by several pharmaceutical brands as a substance which is used to boost the immune system. It can strengthen the capillaries or the tiny blood vessels that carry oxygen and other necessary nutrients to all parts of the body via the bloodstream. It also helps deal with harmful oxygen molecules that could damage the cells in its role as a potent antioxidant. It is also believed that Vitamin C helps maintain cellular health and prevent cancer and a host of other health problems.

Individuals who want to Vitamin C supplementation should seek the recommendation of doctors and other health professionals to side effects and drug interaction. Most people may take up to 2000 mg of Vitamin C without ill effects while some can develop diarrhea from as little as 500 milligrams. It is also important to drink plenty of water because Vitamin C needs to be dissolved in order to be metabolized properly. Sufficient water may also ensure that excess Vitamin C is eliminated from the body.

The reason why Vitamin C is so commonly used in cold and flu medication is because it helps to get rid of toxins in the body known as free radicals. Vitamin C also reduces inflammation and will significantly reduce the severity and duration of the cold.

Vitamin C is commonly known as the following:

- L-ascorbic acid
- Ascorbate

In the body Vitamin C is used to maintain the structure of cells in the form of collagen. It is also used to help with the metabolism of protein and certain neurotransmitters in the brain. Collagen is the form of protein which keeps the skin soft and elastic, removing the appearance of fine lines and wrinkles.

An excess of Vitamin C is extremely hard if not impossible due to the fact that excess Vitamin C is excreted easily from the body in your urine. Usually the only major symptom that an excess of Vitamin C causes is diahorrea.

A deficiency of Vitamin C was historically renowned as scurvy which was prominent amongst the population which sailed on ships for long periods of time. Scurvy occurs when there is an acute lack of Vitamin C such as less than 10mg of Vitamin C per day for a month. Initial symptoms can be fatigue, lack of wound healing, inflammation of the gums and joint pain. Today a deficiency of Vitamin C is very rare in developed countries as we have access to many fruits and vegetables which contain adequate amounts of Vitamin C.

DAILY RECOMMENDED DOSE: 75 mg

Vitamin C is essential for maintaining glowing skin and strong nails. It helps with the production of collagen which is responsible for keeping your skin taut and firm. Collagen is the natural filler your body makes for your skin. Vitamin C also helps in the decrease of free radicals in skin cells, helping to keep them new and youthful looking. Vitamin C will also help to improve the amount of collagen production and result to a more youthful and hydrated looking skin.

This vitamin inhibits the production of melanin, the pigment that gives the skin its dark color and can be used to help ease sign of sunburn or excessive tanning.

Getting rid of free radicals in the body has many good effects. It slows down the aging of the entire body and can help reduce incoming damage that the skin may receive from the sun. So not only does it help to reverse aging, it also puts a stop to any further damage to other systems in the body.

The current recommended daily allowance (RDA) for Vitamin C is 75 milligrams (mg) a day for women and 90 mg a day for men to get the minimum amount the human body needs. However, medical specialists suggest that an intake of 200 mg is accepted since that amount is the most the human body can absorb at one time.

Thankfully so many fruits and veggies are bursting with Vitamin C that you do not need to take this as a supplement. Even an orange per day is enough to fulfill your daily intake. If not, then a cup of broccoli or red pepper can do the trick for you.

Tips when using Vitamin C

Vitamin C should be put on before your sunblock as it will help to quickly eliminate any free radicals that may be caused from ultraviolet (UV) rays which pass through the sunblock. Remember sunscreen can only prevent a certain amount of UV damage.

You should also try to use Vitamins C and E together. Usually they will be found in moisturizers and other skin products together. This is due to the fact that when they synergize together they can be up to 4 times more effective in protecting the skin against free radicals.

Vitamin D

For women Vitamin D is magic. It cuts down on your risk of breast cancer and helps in preventing diabetes and ovarian cancer. For women who work out this is a necessity as Vitamin D is also responsible for muscle function.

Vitamin D can be known as any of the following:

- Drisdol (Vitamin D2)
- Ergocalciferol (Vitamin D2)
- Cholecalciferol (Vitamin D3)

A lack of Vitamin D is rare as our bodies make it while we are out in the sun. The recent studies show that you only need about 10 to 15 minutes of sunlight in order to get your recommended daily dosage. This may include things like walking outside to the post-box or even sitting in the car.

Recent studies have shown support for Vitamin D as a beneficial vitamin that is also beneficial in fighting infections.

It is important to note that the form of Vitamin D that is in supplements and the Vitamin D that our bodies produce naturally with exposure to the sun are two different forms. However their functionality is the same.

The Institute of Food and Agricultural Sciences (IFAS) reports new intake recommendations (based on international units — IUs — per day). These figures are less than previously recommended.

- Children and teens: 600 IU
- Adults up to age 70: 600 IU
- Adults over age 70: 800 IU
- Pregnant or breastfeeding women: 600 IU

This is the one Vitamin that you will need supplements for if you lack exposure to sunlight however Vitamin D supplementation should be monitored by a health professional. Items like milk, salmon and orange juice do have traces of Vitamin D, but it is not enough.

Vitamin E

Oxygen is one of the primary components of nature that supports life. However the same oxygen, when metabolized in the body through certain molecules can become overly reactive and start to cause damage through the formation of free radicals. This normal metabolic process is called oxidative stress. Vitamin E, as an antioxidant, helps prevent oxidative stress, thereby preventing cell damage and aging of the cells.

When the body absorbs cholesterol it is transferred from the liver to other areas to be stored as fat. They are carried in the bloodstream in a small package by a molecule called Low Density Lipoproteins (LDL). When LDL gets oxidized, they react with cholesterol and a waxy fat substance called plaque is deposited on the walls of the arteries, which results in the stopping of blood flow, high blood pressure and cardio-vascular diseases.

Vitamin E helps prevent the conversion of cholesterol into plaque, and this is done by alpha-tocopherol, not any other form of Vitamin E, because liver places it preferentially in the bloodstream through a protein called alpha-tocopherol transfer protein.

The effect of Vitamin E in preventing cancer has not conclusively been established. According to a study by The American Association of Cancer Research, there is a reduced risk of cancer is associated with an intake of Vitamin E-rich foods. However, a study done by Iowa Women's Health Study finds little evidence that Vitamin E has protective effect against breast cancer in women after menopause. Hence, researchers have noted that not just vitamin E alone, but foods rich in antioxidants may be able to protect from cancer.

Numerous studies have established the effect of Vitamin E in protecting the skin from ultraviolet radiation, whose harmful effects include photodermatitis, an allergic type reaction to the UV rays of the sun. Vitamin E, whether taken through foods or applied topically, has been shown to protect skin cell membranes.

Besides these benefits, Vitamin E may protect from Alzheimer's, cataracts (clouding of the lens of the eyes), and pancreatitis (inflammation of the pancreas). Also, Vitamin E may be beneficial in healing wounds and burns, reducing scars. The property of combating oxidative stress may be useful for athletes, as their oxygen utilization rate is higher than those not doing exercise, which results in increased generation of free radicals which can cause visible signs of aging.

Foods such as tofu, spinach and nuts are rich in Vitamin E.

The B-complex vitamins, made simple

The B group of vitamins may be one of the most commonly misunderstood of the vitamins; simply because these are several distinct vitamins lumped together. The fact that the vitamins in this group are known by both letter and number becomes confusing to many people. It's just often more difficult to remember numbers, meaning you may remember that it's one of the "B vitamins," but not remember which number is associated with that particular one. It may help to find out that each of the B vitamins also has a name.

- B1 is also thiamine

- B2 is also riboflavin

- B3 is also niacin

- B5 is also pantothenic acid

- B6 is also pyridoxine

- B7 is also biotin

- B9 is also folic acid

- B12 is also cobalamin

You should note that there are four additional substances in the B complex group, though they are not known as vitamins because they are not necessary for normal body function. They are choline, lipoic acid, PABA and inositol. When you purchase B complex vitamins, these four will not be included, and at least one or two of the recognized B vitamins may also be omitted. B5 and B7 are so widely available in food that most people simply get enough of these vitamins, even if they aren't eating a healthy diet.

Arguably one of the most commonly recognized uses of the B vitamins is an energy booster. Some health care professionals tout the advantages of taking B12 in large doses to combat tiredness, but most seem to agree that starting a regimen of B vitamins is only advisable in severe cases.

More recently, research suggests that some Vitamin B deficiencies may aggravate certain health issues or health risks, and that an increase of those vitamins will help relieve symptoms or lessen the risk. Notably, Alzheimer's is one of those diseases and sufferers of this disease sometimes show improvement from added Vitamin B on a daily basis. Vitamin B2 has also been used to help some migraine patients.

The correlation between certain health issues and vitamin deficiencies is certain; though finding the right treatment may be tricky. One of the most common problems with using vitamins from the B complex group to treat health issues is the fact that many diseases and health issues have overlapping symptoms. Treating those symptoms may ultimately cause more problems than it cures. Talk to your health care professional before taking extraordinary steps toward a vitamin regimen, including those that include complex B vitamins.

Vitamin B1

Vitamin B1 is commonly known as thiamine and can be found in a large array of foods such as yeast, cereal, beans, nuts and meat. It is necessary for the body to be able to break down and utilize carbohydrates.

For adults the RDA is about 1-2mg of thiamine.

A deficiency has been associated with Wernicke-Korsakoff syndrome, caused by alcoholism which causes the depletion of Vitamin B1 in the brain.

It is usually only taken as a supplement on its own if there is a sever deficiency of it such as in beriberi, and inflammation of the nerves (neuritis) associated with pellagra or pregnancy. It can also be used to aid with digestion, helping increase the immune response for those suffering with AIDS, vision problems, motion sickness, and the progression of kidney disease in people with type 2 diabetes.

Vitamin B2

Vitamin B2 (riboflavin), as with all the other B vitamins is essential for energy production in the body however it is used both in the electron transport chain and in the metabolism of fat into energy. B2 is also used in converting other B vitamins into compounds which can be used in the body.

B2 is also used to help recycle a compound called glutathione in the body. Glutathione is an antioxidant responsible for cleaning up free radicals which damage your DNA.

Foods such as spinach, maple syrup, peppers, beet greens and broccoli are all rich in Vitamin B2.

Vitamin B2 loses its potency in the light, which is why milk cartons and other dairy products which have Vitamin B2 are packed in paper or opaque packaging. Even some light exposure will make the B2 to degrade, giving your milk a less fresh taste. Despite this, Vitamin B2 is extremely stable against heat and refrigeration.

The RDI for Vitamin B2 is 1.7mg per 2000 calories consumed.

Vitamin B3

Niacin (Vitamin B3) is useful for the regulation of fats in the body. Several studies have shown that it can boot levels of good HDL cholesterol and lower triglycerides which are our short term reserve of fat. It is for this reason that Niacin is used in combination with cholesterol-lowering medications. However, on its own Niacin is only good for lowering cholesterol in dangerously high doses which need to be prescribed and overseen by a health professional.

Fish, chicken and turkey have the highest quantities of Vitamin B3.

Vitamin B5 (Pantothenic Acid)

The B5 vitamin is one of the most prolific of all the vitamins and can be found in various types of foods. In fact, it is almost impossible for a person to consume less B5 vitamin than they need. For this reason, there is actually no recommended daily amount that health professionals can state as everyone obtains more than enough from their normal food consumption.

Even though there is no need to calculate the recommended daily allowance it does not mean that Vitamin B5 is not needed. In fact, the B5 vitamin is essential for turning food into energy amongst many other roles in the human body. The B5 vitamin is responsible for taking the fats and carbohydrates into energy through different chemical reactions.

The B5 vitamin works in conjunction with other B vitamins especially thiamine or B1, riboflavin or B2, niacin or B3, pyridoxine or B6, and biotin. Along with these other B vitamins, the B5 vitamin is an integral part in a number of processes for maintaining constant energy production. The most important role of B5 is to produce energy from food that is consumed via a metabolic pathway known as the Krebs cycle.

Some B5 vitamin can be found in almost every food whether it is animal or vegetable. Of course there are some sources of the B5 vitamin that are better than others however a balanced and nutritious diet will provide more than enough. The foods with the highest B5 vitamin content are organ meats, salmon, eggs, beans, milk, and whole grains. It is worth noting that the B5 vitamin is lost when grains are milled into flour and tends not to be added back in. Therefore, processed grain foods such as bread, pasta, breakfast cereal, and baked goods are not good sources of the B5 vitamin.

B5 is also extremely helpful in alleviating the symptoms of stress. This is chiefly due to the fact that during periods of stress, the body produces increased adrenalin and this requires the B5 vitamin. There are no known adverse effects to consuming too much B5 vitamin.

Vitamin B6

When most people hear the word "anemia," they immediately think of iron. But a shortage of Vitamin B6 can also cause a type of anemia because this vitamin is vital to the healthy generation of hemoglobin in the blood of a normal, healthy person. You may also associate Vitamin B6 with sugar diabetes, and that's because one of the important functions of this vitamin is to regulate the amount of sugar in the blood.

Vitamin B6 is also known as pyridoxine. You may not have heard of many people who were found to have a serious Vitamin B6 deficiency, and there's a good reason for that. B6 is so readily available in so many foods that it's a fairly simple matter to get your daily recommended allowances of this vitamin.

Some of the common sources of B6 include tuna, roast beef, tomato juice, trout, pork loin and peanut butter. Naturally, cereals that are fortified with vitamins are excellent sources and many provide 100% of the body's need for cereal. Three raw bananas also provide a full day's supply of the necessary Vitamin B6. A medium baked potato (including the potato skin) provides about one-third of the daily requirement. Evaluating the foods rich in this vitamin reveals that many people are already meeting the daily requirements for B6.

So what are the dangers of having too little Vitamin B6 in your daily diet? Recent studies suggest that a lack of this vitamin is a factor for determining the risk of stroke and some types of heart disease. That means that people with deficiencies are more likely to suffer from these health issues than their counterparts who are getting sufficient amounts of Vitamin B6.

Depression is another problem potentially impacted by a Vitamin B6 deficiency. Though there may be some difference of opinion as to the role and the importance of B6 and depression, there appears to be a link that can't be denied. In fact, depression is listed by some as one of the symptoms of insufficient Vitamin B6 in the diet.

There are some risks of taking too much B6. Nerves – especially in the outer extremities – are sometimes damaged by overdosing the body on vitamin B6. In the majority of cases, simply eliminating any vitamin supplements appears to eliminate the nerve problems as well. It's unlikely that a normal person can take in enough Vitamin B6 from a normal diet to cause toxicity at this level, and more likely that these severe effects of too much B6 are caused by taking too many vitamin supplements containing B6.

Vitamin B12

Vitamin B12 is commonly found in meat and dairy products.

During the last years the vital importance of vitamin B12 and folate for our health has become more obvious. Perhaps you have heard that folate is important during pregnancy. Deficiency can cause severe damages to the fetus. In the USA and other countries one has added synthetic folate to prevent damages to the fetus.

Also B12 is of importance in conjunction with folate as both interact to have an effect. Both vitamins have great importance even in other cases. The risk of developing dementia is for example bigger if you suffer from a deficiency of one of these vitamins.

Vitamin B12 and folate are important for every cell of the body. B12 and folate interact in vital functions of all cells. For example they are necessary for the cells to divide and grow in a normal way. That is why they are of great importance for the growing fetus.

The first symptoms of deficiency can also come from the cells that divide too fast, for example blood cells and the cells of mucous membrane. The symptoms will result in a type of anemia often combined with a read tongue and shear mucous membranes in the mouth.

Both vitamins are also necessary for the nerve system to function well, for the nerve cells and for the signal substances that transmit the nerve impulses. If not treated this kind of deficiency can cause permanent damage of the nerves.

A deficiency may occur as a result of an inability to absorb B12 from food and in strict vegetarians who do not consume any animal foods. As a general rule, most individuals who develop a vitamin B12 deficiency have an underlying stomach or intestinal disorder that limits the absorption of Vitamin B12. Sometimes the only symptom of these intestinal disorders is subtly reduced cognitive function resulting from early B12 deficiency. Anemia and dementia follow later.

Characteristic signs, symptoms and health problems associated with B12 deficiency include anemia, fatigue, weakness, constipation, loss of appetite and weight loss.

Deficiency can also lead to neurological changes such as numbness and tingling in the hands and feet. Additional symptoms of B12 deficiency are difficulty in maintaining balance, depression, confusion, dementia, poor memory and soreness of the mouth or tongue.

Many of these symptoms are very general and can result from a variety of medical conditions other than Vitamin B12 deficiency. It is important to have a physician evaluate these symptoms so that appropriate medical care can be given.

Do You Need Antioxidant Vitamins?

Many food items are antioxidants. These are the foods that have Vitamin A, C and E. These antioxidants vitamins appear to play a role in the body's cell protection system by neutralizing highly reactive molecules that the human body produces. It is natural for our bodies to produce these toxins, and that is why antioxidants are so vital to maintaining the integrity of the cells.

The antioxidants found in fruits, vegetables, teas and supplements are proving to be powerful agents in the fight against disease causing free radicals.

However, in recent years, research has shown that Vitamins taken in higher doses can prevent other chronic diseases like cancer and heart disease. A debate still rages, but there is a plethora of research being done on Vitamin A, C, E, the antioxidant vitamins.

A National Institute of Health clinical trial involving people at high risk of developing advanced stages of Age-related Macular Degeneration (AMD), showed that patients' risk decreased by 25% when treated with high doses of antioxidant vitamins and Zinc.

Another study at the Centre for Disease Control and Prevention (CDC) in Atlanta showed that taking Vitamin E along with multivitamins reduced risk from stroke and heart illness. Among patients who took the combination, mortality risk decreased by 15% for these two diseases.

The National Institutes of Health (NIH) concluded a study suggesting that Vitamin C may fight cancer. They found that in a laboratory setting, high doses of Vitamin C injected directly into the bloodstream killed cancer cells.

Vitamin A, another antioxidant helps build and strengthen bones, tissue, skin and mucous membranes.

Be careful when purchasing vitamins and supplements though. Research has shown that vitamins without their co-factors can almost be useless. Nutrition is a complex process of thousands of chemical reactions within our bodies. Vitamins are always better in their natural state - in the foods we eat, as they also come along with micro nutrients needed for their optimal use in the body. Supplements should never be used in place of a poor diet.

The smart choice is to look for whole food vitamins to supplement an already well-balanced for the times you can't get everything you need at meal time.

Our bodies produce free radicals when we break down food, or exposed to smoking (active or passive) and radiation. Therefore the amount of free radicals our bodies make also depends on our environment.

As free radicals they disrupt and shred important cell structures like the membrane for example. It is the job of antioxidants to rip away their destructive strength. This way the risk of potential chronic illness lowers and in the same way, the aging process does too. Some researchers claim that antioxidants boost the immune system when you are under stress.

Other naturally occurring antioxidants include tannins, phenol, flavonoids and lignans. These are mainly found in plant based foods such as red peppers, broccoli and apricots.

Unfortunately, many adults have trouble getting the right amount of antioxidants in their daily diet. You need to make sure that you get at least five servings of fruits and vegetables in order to keep up with this quota.

Best Sources of Antioxidants

There is a wide and varied list of foods which contains many of the aforementioned antioxidants. This list is not exhaustive at all but is a start on which foods you should be looking out for in order to incorporate antioxidants into your diet.

Berries: Blackberries, blueberries, cranberries, strawberries, and raspberries.

Stone fruits: Peaches, prunes, nectarines, plums, cherries, and apricots

Tropical fruits: Kiwi, mango, banana, pineapple and papaya

Pears and many apple varieties (with peel)

Vegetables: Okra, bell peppers, Artichokes and kale

Sweet potatoes, red and russet potatoes — with the skin on

Nuts: Pistachios, walnuts, hazelnuts almonds and pecans

Legumes: kidney beans, edamame and lentils

Alliums: Onions, shallots, Garlic, Leeks

Certain drinks: Pomegranate juice, tea and coffee as well as the occasional red wine.

Skin Deep

Is the peel or skin as it is better known as, worth keeping on your foods and vegetables?

There have been numerous studies done about the benefits of eating the peel of certain fruits. While it is beneficial and does contain extra fibre and nutrients it is not such a massive amount that getting rid of it will greatly diminish its nutritional benefit.

Therefore if removing the peel makes it more pleasant for you to eat the fruit or vegetable then it is better to remove the peel then to not eat the fruit or vegetable at all.

Remedy for Allergies

Did you know that allergies are a caused by your immune system reacting too much to things that are not harmful to your body? It is true that both genetics and your surroundings are a huge factor when it comes to an over sensitive immune system which results in itching, swelling, rashes, coughing and muscle spasms, leaving the sufferer feeling weak and tired.

You could simply just avoid whatever it is that you are allergic to, but that would be very difficult if you are allergic to something like dust or pollen. You can't avoid these things in daily life. If you did it would be a great inconvenience to you daily activities.

Allergies can also manifest on your skin, causing redness, swelling and even acne. The following is a list of different factors which may trigger your allergies.

Pollen, Dust Mites and Mould

These are well-known for causing allergies. Things like seasonal changes, temperature and how often you wash your sheets will all determine how much exposure you get to these. If pollen levels are high such as during pollination seasons you will be more likely to suffer from allergies. Keeping a clean house and washing yourself after being outside will help to eliminate prolonged exposure to these substances.

Genetics

There is a large amount of evidence to show that you are more predisposed to allergies if it runs in your family. Unfortunately there isn't much you can do about your genetics however keeping healthy and fit will help to alleviate the severity at which you will experience your allergies.

Low Immune System

A weak immune system means that you will not be able to fight off the allergens which will attack your system. Immunity in humans may be weak for several reasons. First, if you do not get enough vitamins and minerals from supplements or a well-balanced diet your immune system will lose its strength and will become less effective in fighting allergens and other forms of viruses or infections.

Your immune system will also take a huge hit if you are prone to mental stress. This can make you physically weak as hormones produced in the body when you are stressed actively suppress the immune system. To strengthen your immune system make sure you get lots of vitamins, eat a healthy diet and avoid stress as much as possible.

Many studies have been done and there has been no discovery yet to show if there is a singular factor that causes allergies. Allergies can be caused by one of the reasons listed above or possibly a combination of many different reasons. Keeping up a healthy lifestyle by exercising, sleeping and eating healthy will help alleviate the symptoms of allergies by keeping your immune system strong.

Luckily most of the foods that you need to help diminish you allergy problems are available at your local supermarket. You need to start looking for foods rich in Vitamin C and Omega 3 fatty acids.

Vitamin C is undoubtedly one of the best things to come out of nature. It's a natural antihistamine and functions by killing the molecular form of histamine. The absorption greatly depends on the amount consumed. Therefore it is recommended that you take more than 500 milligram daily through either supplements or food.

Eating fruits rich in Vitamin C cut down on asthma symptoms in kids around the age of 8. Moreover it has also been proven that when you take bioflavins along with Vitamin C you can actually benefit from enhanced Vitamin C. Bioflavonoids can be naturally found in rosehip. Remember if you are taking Vitamin C from a natural source then you should eat them fresh; storing Vitamin C or having it exposed to air will make it lose its potency.

For Stretch Marks

Around 70% of women develop stretch marks during pregnancy. The best part is that these become less noticeable 6 months or a year after the pregnancy. Stretch marks are pink, purple, dark brown or purple depending on your skin color. Over time they usually fade to a light grey or brown color.

Stretch Marks Caused by Pregnancy

Women develop stretch marks during pregnancy from the skin stretching on the abdomen and the breasts as they grow in size rapidly to accommodate for the growing fetus. Stretch marks can also be a result of hormonal changes inside the body. What happens is that hormones attract water to the skin and that makes the collagen fibers relax. This increased fragility in the structure makes it very easy for the skin to get damaged.

It is literally impossible to predict who won't suffer from stretch marks during pregnancy and who will. However, researchers claim that genes play a huge part in this. For instance if your sister or mother had stretch marks during pregnancy then chances are strong that you will have them too. Plus other studies show that young women like teen moms are more prone to them. Moreover you are also likely to have bigger stretch marks if you gain weight fast, if you are carrying more than one baby and if you have excess amniotic fluid.

When you adopt a healthy diet during pregnancy then it only makes sense that you will gain weight rapidly. During the pregnancy eating things like supplements and foods rich in Vitamin E like sunflowers, blueberries, almonds and papaya can aid in actually preventing the appearance of stretch marks. However if you are struggling to eat Vitamin E rich foods everyday then supplements can aid in reaching the daily recommended intake. It is important to keep in mind that supplements should not be a complete substitute for a healthy balanced diet.

We often hear about skin creams and expensive laser treatments that claim to remove stretch marks but these methods have risks associate with them and can be very costly. Therefore it is recommended that pregnant women apply Vitamin E oil onto the body parts which are most likely to develop stretch marks; for instance the area around the stomach. Vitamin E helps the skin to become softer, allowing it to stretch without causing bruising in the skin which creates stretch marks.

Other than the fact that taking Vitamin E helps improve the strength and elasticity of your skin; it also helps ease the appearance of lines and wrinkles. Basically Vitamin E works to gather the epidermis and then acts as a shield against evaporation of moisture. This way the skin remains hydrated.

Plus if you have had surgery healthy doses of Vitamin E can speed up the healing process. You have to take it for a month before the surgery and after it to work though. It can also improve the appearance of scars, surgical or otherwise.

Stretch Marks Outside of Pregnancy.

Sometimes women may have genetically fibrous skin. This mean that during times of rapid growth, such as accelerated weight gain or growth spurts at puberty the body grows faster than the skin can handle causing stretch marks to occur.

The type of skin that is prone to stretch marks is genetic and therefore cannot be helped. There is however treatments that can reduce the appearance of them as discussed above.

Heal and Rejuvenate Your Skin

You probably already know that there are three basics to having a beautiful and glowing skin: don't smoke, protect your skin from UV rays and eat healthy. But not many people are aware that antioxidants and vitamins can greatly make a difference to your skin as well.

Shield from the Sun

Researchers have discovered that Vitamins E and C are effective in protecting the skin from the harmful rays of the sun. This way they also lower your chances of skin cancer. These anti-oxidants function by accelerating the skin's natural repair system. If you must take supplements it is recommended that you take 1000 to 3000 milligrams of Vitamin C with 400 IU of Vitamin E. Remember for good skin you can mix this up with 100 to 200 micrograms of selenium.

Protect From Cancer

Another natural antioxidant in the body is the Coenzyme Q10 which helps the cells grow and protects them from the ravages of cancer. A fall in the levels of coenzyme Q10 occurs as we age and it shows in our skin. Therefore the use of this natural antioxidant can minimize the appearance of wrinkles. So far studies have only been able to record results of 0.3% concentration or more of it.

Alpha Lipoic for Skin Damage

Alpha Lipoic Acid is another antioxidant which is used topically. The cream is great for protecting the skin from sun damage. Studies have found great improvement in skin if around 4% concentration of the Alpha Lipoic Acid is present in the cream and if it is used every other day.

Fountain of Youth

Retinoic Acid is sort of an active type of Vitamin A inside the skin and also dubbed the best when it comes to anti-ageing. You can use topical retinoic acid for age spots, wrinkles and the rough damage caused by the sun. Basically Retinoic Acid helps restore the elasticity in the skin. But you must not use it too must as it can result in peeling, redness and dryness of the skin. Dermatologists recommend that you start with a small concentration; we are talking from 0.01% tot no more than 0.1% and apply it after every two nights.

Chocolate and Green Tea

Did you know that chocolate and green teas are good for your skin? Green tea harbors flavonoids that are very strong and may help protect the skin from cancer and inflammation. A German study experimented with women drinking hot cocoa with a great concentration of flavonoid for 90 days; the result was softer and much smoother skin by the end of the study period. Another study found that women whose skin was treated with green tea extract had lesser risks of incurring skin damage after exposure to sun light.

We already have established that B Vitamins are great for the entire human body. It is important to consume foods that are rich in these to get great looking skin. Start eating chicken, eggs and whole grains to gain its benefits.

It would be wise of you stopped believing all the hype that companies create about how their products can give miraculous results. When a product simply claims that it includes Vitamins C or E you don't know exactly how much the quantity is and therefore you cannot tell whether using that product would be beneficial to you or not. Sometimes the amounts may be extremely minimal and not beneficial to you at all.

There are guidelines in certain countries, such as Australia which demand that all notable ingredient and nutrients be recorded on the packaging however this is not the case for all countries that are able to put labels on their food with minimal testing of their nutritional content.

For Healthy Eyes

Many of us try to eat the sort of foods that would slim us down but in the process we are forgetting about other important things that we should be taking care of in our bodies, such as our eyes, skin and nails.

Our eyes are a very important indicator of our health. They can show whether or not you have certain health issues such as copper deficiency, or if you are sleep deprived. Having healthy eyes that are bright and clear is a sign of good health.

The truth is that Vitamins provide you with overall wellness and in the same way their deficiency can cause health related problems for you. The three Vitamins that are vital for eye health are Vitamin A, C and E.

In general Vitamin A is a group of antioxidant compounds. This compound aids in building the immune system, bone strength and good vision. Vitamin A works to make healthy the mucous membrane (around the eye and the skin. If there is a defect in this layer then Bacteria and viruses can easily attack and pose infections, respiratory illnesses etc.)

That Vitamin A that comes from animal derived edibles is referred to as retinol. This form of Vitamin A can be directly digested by the human body.

On the other hand the Vitamin A that is taken from fruits and veggies are what we commonly known as Provitamin A carotenoids. These when consumed are changed into retinol by the body.

What Does Vitamin A Do For Our Eyes?

We already established that Vitamin A helps protect the surface of the eye i.e. the cornea and boosts vision.

Vitamin A eye drops have been effective for treating a certain type of eye inflammation known as superior limbic keratoconjunctivitis.

When Vitamin A is combined with other antioxidant Vitamins it also helps reducing the risk of macular degeneration.

In addition to that a combination of Vitamin A and lutein may be the cause of prolonging eye vision for victims of retinitis pigmentosa. A recent study found that people with this disease once they took supplements of lutein and vitamin A everyday lost their peripheral vision much later than the individuals who did not take the supplements.

Beta Carotene, the form that it is usually found in within food, is converted into Vitamin A once it enters the body and because of that the benefits of taking it are a lot similar to that of retinol.

Not Enough Vitamin A

Vitamin A deficiency is not that common in developed countries. It is however very common in many developing countries. It is said that that malnourished children become blind on a global scale. This is due to Vitamin A deficiency. A lack of Vitamin A makes the cornea get really dry. It continues with the clouding of the front of the eye and then vision loss.

Is Vitamin A All You Need For Good Vision?

Vitamin C seems to creep its way into every health and beauty benefit there is. You can find it in strawberries, kiwi, grapefruit, oranges, peppers, broccoli and mustard greens. In addition to providing antioxidants to the body it also helps in slowing down cataracts and macular degeneration.

Vitamin E is a great antioxidant and also shields the eye from macular degeneration and cataracts. You will find Vitamin E in several nuts such as pine nuts, pea nuts and almond. Vitamin E is also found in sunflower seeds and dried apricots.

All this shows us that consuming the correct amounts of Vitamins on a daily basis earlier in life can be all the defense you need against preventable vision problems that creep up later in life. No matter what your age you can always start by eating fruits and vegetables today.

Food for Gorgeous and Healthy Eyes

- Carrots have Beta carotenes are important for maintaining healthy eyes. Most of the foods that are orange in color have beta carotene, which is the element which gives them their color hue.
- Leafy greens have lutein and zeaxanthin: these are antioxidants that reduce the risk of cataracts and macular degeneration over time.
- Eggs are a source of zinc, lutein and zeaxanthin. They also aid in cutting down the risk of macular degeneration.
- Berries are packed with Vitamin C.
- Almonds have lots of Vitamin E. One handful each day can provide half of your daily intake.
- Anchovies, trout, salmon, mackerel and tuna all have DHA which is a fatty acid that is present in your retina. Low DHA is linked to dry eye syndrome.

Skin Allergies

A simple but effective way to manage skin allergies is through this 3 step approach. Firstly you must understand the condition, and then discover if anything is triggering your skin reaction, and thirdly looking after you allergy-prone skin.

When we think of allergies, we usually think about respiratory or digestive problems however allergies frequently affect the largest organ in the body, your skin. As with other allergies the immune system overreacts to the presence of certain substances and releases inflammation-producing chemicals. Do some research and talk to your doctor. You can be confident of controlling your skin condition better if you are sure you understand what causes it.

The second component in managing a skin allergy is identifying then eliminating the allergens and irritants that start the itching/scratching cycle. There are over three thousand known triggers for skin allergies. Many are natural, but there are plenty of man-made ones too.

A common man-made trigger is latex, which comes from the sap of the Brazilian rubber tree. The natural proteins and those added in the manufacturing process can trigger an allergic reaction. Most people are aware that this can lead to reactions if you wear latex gloves. However latex is also present in baby pacifiers, balloons, pencil erasers and elastic bands in undergarments. There can also be problems when latex particles become airborne and are inhaled. If you have latex allergy try to avoid the material and use vinyl or plastic where possible.

Nickel is another common trigger of skin allergies. In addition to the obvious nickel-containing metallic objects like coins and jewelry, nickel is also present in everyday objects like scissors, bathroom and kitchen cabinet handles, and zippers. Mascara, eye shadow and eye pencils also contain trace amounts of nickel. Studies have given an estimate that the number of people suffering from a nickel allergy has raised to about 40% in the last decade. Much of this is believed to be due to the popularity of body piercing which has become more common.

Foods also have natural nickel content and people who suffer severe symptoms may need to restrict their diet under medical supervision if they are particularly sensitive to nickel. At present there is no way to desensitize a person with a nickel allergy. Avoidance is the best strategy.

The third component of effective management is looking after your skin. A simple but effective way to help is to cut your nails to ease the skin thickening caused by excessive scratching.

Managing your skin's condition means firstly moisturizing and softening the skin to ensure it does not dry out. Your doctor may recommend you use topical corticosteroid preparations to control the inflammation.

When you take a bath soak in lukewarm water for 20 to 30 minutes. Do not have hot baths or showers, as the heat will increase skin dryness and itching. You can add oatmeal or baking soda to the bath for a soothing effect, though it does not help moisturize the skin.

Use a mild soap or a non-soap cleanser with neutral pH (pH7). If you wish to add bath oils do so after you have been in the water so that it can seal in the moisture. Do not use bubble baths as they can form a barrier that stops the bathwater moisturizing your skin.

After the bath dry yourself by patting your skin with a soft towel. This helps retain moisture. Immediately after drying your skin apply a lotion or emollient cream to help your skin retain the moisture.

To look after your skin you will also need to avoid situations where you will experience extreme physical contact, heavy perspiration, or heavy clothing. This may mean avoiding some sports. Swimming is permissible if you rinse the chlorine from your skin as soon as you leave the pool, and use a moisturizer after drying yourself.

Follow these three steps and you will be able to control your skin allergy and minimize its impact on your everyday life.

Sunburn

At some time or another, we've all experienced the effects of sunburn whether it is either mild or severe. Even those with darker shades of skin can get sunburn, however they will be less likely to peel and show the other signs of sunburn such as erythema (redness of the skin).

Although the sting of regret of inadequate protection (from UV exposure) can be an excellent incentive to plan more carefully on 'future' occasions, it's of little help in soothing the immediate physical sting (i.e. pain) accompanying sunburn.

However if you have found yourself having spent a little too much time in the sun, -- here are 4 natural home remedies to help ease the pain of sunburn, and assist in the body's healing process:

1. Cool Milk Compresses: - The fat and lactic acids in milk are known to have soothing qualities for sunburned skin. Soak a soft cloth or cotton gauze in cool whole milk, and dab carefully onto the burned skin. Do this for around 20 minutes, and follow by rinsing off with cool water. (Due to the importance of the milk's fat content, it's important that whole milk be used in this treatment).

2. Cool, sugarless tea: - The tannin in tea is the active ingredient here, which helps to soothe and relieve some of the discomfort of sunburned skin. After brewing a big pot of tea, and allowing it to cool completely, slosh the affected areas with a soft sponge or washcloth. You could also fill a spray bottle, and spray the tea directly on the skin. And don't throw away the used (cool) teabags. These are especially good for sensitive areas around the eyes – simply place the teabags over your eyes if they feel hot and tired.

3. Aloe Vera: - Aloe Vera is commonly used to treat sunburn. As well as providing soothing relief, it may also assist in the healing process. Apply to the affected areas as needed. Although the gel extracted directly from an aloe Vera plant works best, if you don't have ready access to one, you may use an 'over the counter' Aloe Vera Cream that contains the gel. For this to be effective, just ensure that the cream contains a high concentration of Aloe Vera than it does water or other solutions.

4. Water: - When exposed to the sun, your body loses water and essential body salts. Dehydration occurs when your body loses too much fluid, and begins to reabsorb fluid from the blood and other body tissues. To prevent the consequences of dehydration, increase your fluid intake to ensure you adequately re-hydrate your body for optimum recovery and health.

Sunburn should of course be avoided where possible due to the fact that long term frequent exposure can result in skin cancer. Prevention and protection should always be considered the best treatment for sunburn, and will assist in ensuring your optimum long-term health.

Sensitive Skin

Skin care regimens have different effects on each skin type. This means that skin care treatments and products work well in certain types of skin. Hence, it is really very important for a person to determine his skin type in order to know which products are best on his skin.

Among the five skin types, sensitive skin is probably the hardest type to maintain and handle, for it is more prone to burning, stinging, drying, itching, and other skin complications. People with sensitive skin type also experience adverse reactions with sudden climate changes, certain skin care products, and abrupt feelings of stress.

According to statistics, fair-skinned individuals are usually the ones who have sensitive skin, regardless of ethnic background. In addition to the common complications associated with sensitive skin are a couple of serious skin conditions like eczema, rosacea, and psoriasis.

Sensitive Skin Care Info

Although sensitive skin is the type that is more prone to skin complications, maintaining this skin type is not really that hard once a person learns how to simplify his or her daily skin care routines. It is not really advisable for one to maintain sensitive skin with so many products and treatments, for these will only result to serious irritations and blemishes. Over-washing sensitive skin is also a big no no. Since this type of skin easily reacts with environmental elements, sunscreen is a must in caring and maintaining the skin.

How to Choose the Best Skin Care Product for Sensitive Skin

Today's market offers numerous skin care options for consumers to choose from. The dilemma, however, is how to find the one that best suits a sensitive skin type. Below is a quick guide on how to choose skin care products for sensitive skin:

1.   Look for organic or natural skin care products instead of the conventional ones as these are the best aids for sensitive skin. Organic or natural skin care products do not contain dye or perfume ingredients that are harmful to the skin.

2.   For cleaning sensitive skin, it is best to use a soap-free cleansing product. People with sensitive skin are also encouraged to use skin care products that contain ingredients like salicylic acid if acne still occurs.

3.   Always look for a mild and alcohol-free astringent products for these are also perfect skin care aid for sensitive skin. However, if irritation or redness occurs, immediately discontinue use.

4.   When using or applying make-up, purchase cosmetic products or items that are non-comedogenic and water-based. Although these cosmetics are a bit more expensive, these are safer and milder on the skin, thus, preventing irritation and dryness.

5.   As for moisturizers, those with sensitive skin should go for the products that are fragrance-free and hypoallergenic. Regularly maintaining the skin with moisturizers also prevents aging signs such as wrinkles and facial lines.

Eczema

Eczema is an inflammation of the skin frequently seen in conjunction with allergic conditions such as asthma and hay fever. Unfortunately these make up the triad of familiar genetic conditions seen most commonly in people.

Eczema is extremely uncomfortable and is a chronic condition. The parts affected by eczema develop lesions which will often appear as patches, blisters and scratches. The vicinities affected by eczema are very itchy and uncomfortable. The affected areas may become abnormally thick.

Thickening of the skin can be brought through trauma to the patches from scratching and rubbing. The affected spots will be typically dry in comparison to unaffected areas. The face, elbows, behind the knees, wrists are more likely to develop eczema than other body parts.

One of the major causes of eczema is the imbalance in a person's immune function and is probably a form of response to the environmental substances such as dust, pollution, yeast, cosmetic products, chemicals such as: detergents, oils, greases, solvents at home or in the work place. In addition, stress can cause a depletion of certain body nutrients (vitamins and minerals), which ultimately leads to a sensitivity towards eczema.

Corticoid creams containing hydrocortisone are the most common conventional treatment for eczema. Hydrocortisone is similar to a natural hormone secreted by adrenal gland, which controls the inflammation process and actively participates in the ionic body balance. The hydrocortisone creams are effective for reducing inflammation, swelling, redness and itching thereby allowing the affected area to heal.

In spite of temporarily reducing the effects of eczema, these creams can lead to skin thinning and damaging. At high doses or at low doses for extended time the hydrocortisone can accumulate through the body and induce metabolic changes in salt and water balance, potassium and calcium balance and increases the blood sugar level. The reasons for accumulation are multiple. One important cause is the competition between the naturally secreted hormone and the topical hydrocortisone for the same receptors, which can raise the uncoupled hormone level. Another important cause is the steroid structure of the hormone, which makes elimination through the kidney difficult.

The corticosteroid creams have to be used with a low dose of hormone and for short period of time as sometimes indicated on the label. On the other hand, sudden discontinuation of the corticosteroid cream can lead to the worsening of the eczema.

Herbal therapy is a mild but long lasting alternative for eczema treatment. Many herbs are known for their beneficial qualities in the treatment of eczema such as: Burdock, Calendula, St. John Wort, Chamomile, Chickweed, Yarrow, Nettle, Licorice. They can be used as teas, tinctures or for topical treatment.

Since eczema is a complex skin disease one single herb is not enough to relieve the symptoms of the eczema or eradicate the disease. A complex mixture of beneficial herbs is more likely to succeed in the treatment.

The antioxidant therapy has been successfully used in the prevention and treatment of different skin diseases, which usually are characterized by a high percentage of free radicals at the site of the affected areas. A good example of natural antioxidants is Sea Buckthorn and Grape seed oils. They contain a wide range of antioxidants such as vitamin E, A, C, selenium, beta carotene and anthocyanin's, which can be beneficial in the case of eczema and other skin disorders.

Natural alternative may be longer than the conventional solution for eczema treatment but much safer for the skin and health in general.

For Healthy and Beautiful Hair

Getting the right vitamins for optimal hair growth is very important. There is some evidence from a few small studies that the western diet has changed significantly in the last 20 years and there are certain vitamin and mineral deficiencies likely to be found in a typical Western diet.

There are different ways in which amino acid supplements may act influence the hair follicles. The mineral rich shampoos and vitamin supplements may act directly on hair stimulating or inhibiting growth activity or they may act indirectly through other intermediaries. For example, a vitamin supplement or herb may influence the production of a hormone to which hair follicles are sensitive such as thyroid hormones or androgens. This change in hormone activity in turn may change the activity of the hair follicles.

Some minerals and vitamins can influence the activity levels of another vitamin and minerals. For example, intake of lysine, vitamin B12 and vitamin C help in absorption of other factors like iron. It is worth bearing in mind that the complexity of the body means there are many potential interactions for even the simplest nutrient.

Vitamins for hair & hair growth

Since Vitamin C, helps the absorption of other factors, it is of some significance. Others are of secondary importance to hair growth like vitamin E. Vitamin E is necessary to provide good blood circulation to the scalp by increasing the uptake of oxygen. Not fundamentally required in a hair growth supplement, vitamin E is often present largely because people expect to see it in the ingredients - and the customer is always right!

Other common ingredients like the amino acids - L-Cysteine and L-Methionine are of questionable value. Although they are fundamentally required for good hair growth, even a rather unhealthy diet should provide enough of these amino acids and supplementation is rarely required.

Co-factors and what do they mean?

The supplement industry is worth several billion dollars a year and it is still growing rapidly. Vitamin supplements, mineral supplements and herbal supplements available on net come in all shapes and forms, many of which are specifically advertised to promote healthy hair growth.

These 'vitamin supplements' vitamins are marketed by different names such as liquid vitamin supplements, natural vitamin supplements, daily vitamin supplements, nutritional vitamin supplements and also by such names as mail order vitamin supplements or best vitamins supplements.

But the for the most part, with a few notable exceptions like vitamin A & Folic acid, taking these supplements probably does not harm hair growth. But whether they can really help promote hair growth depends on what the actual cause of the hair loss is and how the supplements or active ingredients in herbs interact with the hair follicles.

Vitamin and herbal supplements

To buy online health supplements or herbal treatment requires you to go for quality. Unfortunately there is no universal method by which quality supplements can be identified. So it is best to depend upon the natural vitamins supplements or fresh foods.

Typically, vitamins and minerals are most concentrated in fresh foods, the older the food is, and the more processed it is, the less nutritious it is. So in principle, the average diet of the early twenty first century may be more deficient in certain nutrients required for healthy hair growth compared to the average diet of the mid to late twentieth century, but it should be emphasized that vitamin and mineral deficiency is still rarely a cause of hair loss.

Hair loss vitamins & minerals

A comprehensive test for vitamin and mineral levels when one or more is suspected as a cause of hair loss would include; serum iron, serum ferritin, and total iron binding capacity, serum zinc. The deficiency which directly affects hair growth can be related to vitamin B subtypes such as biotin, Vitamin B6 and Vitamin B12. You can go for testing for others if they are on offer, but biotin and B6 testing is enough to cover 95% of vitamin deficiencies related to hair loss. And only when such a deficiency is detected by the tests that you need to buy and eat the 'vitamin supplements' vitamins. So the bottom line is that it is better to have the natural supplements through a balanced diet.

How your Hair Grows

Your hair is made of keratin, the same protein that makes up your nails and the outer layer of your skin. The part you see and style is called the hair shaft. It's actually dead tissue made by your hair follicles tiny bulb-like structures beneath your scalp's surface.

Vitamin C

Vitamin C helps boost the immune system if it is taken as an antioxidant. Did you know that it is used in several hair care products too? It is the one Vitamin that will get you the results that you are looking for. For hair care you can also use products that are simply infused with Vitamin C. It is your responsibility to make sure that you get your daily dose so that your hair looks at its best every day. Whole foods are great for this but of you still think that they are not giving you enough of it then you can always go for supplements.

Vitamin A

Vitamin A is a very powerful antioxidant for the body and has many health properties that make it worthwhile. It is very likely that you might end up taking too much Vitamin A. You must go to the doctor and have all your vitamin levels checked to see where you rank. Having too much may counter the good effects of having optimal Vitamin A in your body. It would be much wiser if you go for supplements. If you have issues with your vision or skin you might be in need of Vitamin A.

Vitamin D

Vitamin D aids in healthy follicle growth so you do not want to skip out of this particular vitamin. The only way you can get the most of it is by getting out of the house. That's right, by getting your fair share of exposure of the sun. You do not need too much of it, just enough to have your body synthesizing its own. However in the winter months when you are mostly stuck indoors, it can create a deficiency of Vitamin D in your body. Of course you can always opt for the Vitamin D supplements and the hair care products that promise it as an ingredient but that is nothing compared to what your body can make on its own.

Vitamin E

Vitamin E is a popular Vitamin when it comes to hair care. You can either get the benefit of this Vitamin by consuming foods that have them or by taking multivitamins that harbor them. If formerly you were suffering from severe deficiency then you will see an exponential change in the way your hair looks. Vitamin E when it is combined with other vitamins that help promote healthy hair result in a healthy scalp that boosts hair growth. If you fail to see any improvements by using hair care products that promise this, then start trying to find other sources in your daily diet.

B Vitamins

B Vitamins are always mentioned together because there are tons of these and you will want to cover all of them. You can either eat whole food that are rich in these or simply opt for a B vitamin complex. You can even just buy shampoos and conditioners that have them. Signs of not getting enough B Vitamins include you feeling really weak and tired, getting easily bruised and slow hair growth. For hair care Vitamin B 12 is the best but for really good results try incorporating them, in your daily plan.

Dry Hair

Dry hair occurs mainly due to harsh external factors such as heat, chemicals or just neglect. Everybody's hair has a certain amount of innate moisture which preserves it and does not let it dry. One should keep in mind that excess experiments with your hair such as constant coloring, bleaching or heat treatment can cause problems and lead to dry hair.

Some of the common reason why many face this problem is the excessive washing of your hair. Your hair does not need to be washed daily as this washes out oils and nutrients from your hair leaving it dry and brittle. In addition, use of hot dryers, hot curlers or any heat-based hair styling treatments can lead to drying. Swimming in chlorinated water without a head cap makes your hair parched and even drier. By using some of the home based recipes you can make your last longer with a better look.

The use of mild shampoo is one of the initial steps to be taken when you are treating dry hair. Look for shampoos mentioned as 'dry and damaged' which would work in your favour. The use of conditioner is a must as this helps in preserving the lost nutrients and oil in your hair. This would give a beautiful look to your hair with the extra shine and bounce. Snipping off the end of your hair would help in preventing further damage to your hair. Exposure to sun can also cause dryness. You can use hair sunscreen to protect your hair.

Some homemade treatments can be beneficial for your hair and are easy to use. For example, beer seems to work wonders on your hair. You can spray your hair with beer once you have shampooed your hair. Studies have shown that beer swells the hair cuticles as well as leaving a protective shiny coating on your hair. It is best to use the traditional beer made from hops as it does not contain many of the chemicals that commercial contains which is not good for your body let alone you hair. Mayonnaise is also a wonderful ingredient which brings life back to your hair.

Thinning Hair

We have all heard of someone who has thinning hair problem, but the problem may be more extensive that you think. Some of the statistics below will surprise you.

1. 70 million Americans have fine or thin looking hair with this amount of people constantly increasing.

3. By age 65, 48% of all women report they have thinning hair and 75% of all men report they have noticeably thin-looking hair.

4. Research has shown that the problem of thin-looking hair can begin as early as age 17.

How does hair loss start?

Hair loss is actually a normal symptom of aging and is often non-pathological. As we age, the cells that are responsible for producing hair begin to die and therefore cannot produce as much keratin as needed. 50 to 60 hairs are shed each day from a normal scalp. Losing more than 60 hairs a day is called excessive hair loss and leads to generalized thinning of the hair. Hair becomes fine in texture. Loss of hair in men is often determined by heredity or by the Alopecia Androgenetic hormone. Hair loss in women is often caused by pregnancy, stress, fatigue or medical treatment.

Can Thyroid Disease Cause Hair Loss?

An overactive or underactive thyroid can cause hair loss. One may get her thyroid numbers in order after beginning a regimen of thyroid medication. However, there have been reported cases of women experiencing hair loss as a side effect of thyroid medication.

Ways to help hide thinning hair

Coloring: If you inherited a tendency for hair loss, the hair that you do have will be healthy. Therefore, your hair can benefit from permanent or semi-permanent color to give body and volume to hair.

Volumising Products: Many volume-building hair products contain paraffin, which is beeswax. That's not good for hair, because it builds up and can make hair break.

However, volumising products sold in salons do help. They won't weigh hair down, and they won't damage it. Mousse, for example, can be applied at the root area for support. Then, begin blow-drying the root area, applying tension with a brush to build volume. Use a light finishing spray to hold it.

For Strong and Healthy Nails

What Are Nails Made of?

Nails are made up of keratin and the same protein that is present in nails and hair. Nails do not only need this protein but C, E, A and B Vitamins as well. When our nails do not get enough of these or when our body is not absorbing them due to certain factors like illness or stress. This way your nails will become brittle and dull.

The Vitamins You Need

Everyone knows that in order to have beautiful and healthy nails you need to have proper nutrition, minerals and vitamins. Sometimes you need a little extra help from vitamins or supplements to get super healthy nails. At the same time you also need to make sure that you do not put undue stress on nails by using them as something to pick and pluck with all the time.

Vitamin A helps you grow healthy nails. If you are taking Vitamin Supplements of Vitamin A then do try to avoid taking alcohol and caffeine as they lower that specific Vitamin's levels. This is because they both compete for the same spot of absorption.

Scientists acknowledge that very low levels of Vitamin B can make nails thin and cause them to break. Stack up on your B Vitamins and folic acid the deficiency of which can also pose brittle nails.

Lower levels of Vitamin C are famous for causing Hang Nails. So start eating your Vitamin C's today. Citrus fruit or supplements as discussed earlier can do the trick.

Vitamin E is not just an antioxidant but aids blood circulation which in turn helps nail growth. Apart from consuming Vitamin E make sure that you use nail polish remover with Vitamin E in it that way you will get an extra kick of the vitamin.

Prenatal Vitamins Outside of Pregnancy

Pregnant women experience healthier hair and nails. People think it is because of prenatal Vitamins. It is not! The healthy nails and hair is a result of pregnancy and if you are not pregnant then there is no need to waste your money on extra prenatal vitamins. Your healthy die and Vitamin supplements will do the trick. However if you are pregnant, prenatal Vitamins are exceptionally important and are recommended by National medical agencies around the world.

5 Things Your Nails Trying To Tell You

Did you know that you can tell what Vitamins you need by the look of your nails?

1. Nails that are dry and peel easily are a sign that you are Vitamin C and D deficient.
2. In the same way weal nails are a sign that the body needs zinc, silicon, iron and Vitamin B. When your nails break easily it means that they need protein and B Vitamins.
3. If you experience hang nails frequently then it is a direct sign of Vitamin C and folic acid deficiency.
4. If your nails develop horizontal or vertical ridges then your body needs B vitamins.
5. Some women are prone to having fungus accumulate under their nails for this it is necessary that they take their fair share of B vitamins. In this situation what happens is that your body has very low levels of good bacteria. It usually occurs when you start taking antibiotics on a daily basis.

Without the proper nutrition nails can become compromised and become soft and weak.

Tips for Beautiful Looking Nails

- Do not pick or bite your nails
- Make sure your nails are clean at all times.

- You must put moisturizer to your nails and the cuticles on a daily basis. Creams that have urea, lactic acid and phospoholipids function to shield against cracking.
- Never file your nails to a point. Always file them in a single direction and slightly round the tip.
- Do not cut your nails too deep or too clean that would be an open invitation to infection.
- Never dig out ingrown toenails. If it starts bothering you do not take up a DIY project, instead see a dermatologist.
- When you are purchasing nail polish removers make sure you do not buy ones that have acetone or formaldehyde.
- If you like getting manicures then take your own instruments.
- Women with artificial nails should check regularly for greenish discoloration which is a sign of bacterial infestation.
- Healthy nails and hair are a result of adequate nutrition, vitamins and supplements. If you do not get enough of these then you are surely missing out on things like

Vitamins for Beautiful Teeth

Your body needs a combination of Vitamins and minerals in order to maintain health including your oral health. Vitamins are great for oral health and the best part is that they are easily found in the food and beverages that you take on a daily basis.

Take a look at your average food intake and see for yourself if you are getting enough of the Vitamins that you need.

Vitamin D

Let's start with the most important Vitamin for oral health. Vitamin D helps you absorb calcium. Your teeth and your jawbone also need calcium for good health. People deficient in Vitamin D can suffer from a condition called Burning Mouth Syndrome. The symptoms of this syndrome are: dry mouth, metallic taste and burning sensation. And to add to that dry mouth can most likely cause tooth decay because of imbalanced saliva levels which secrete to balance the acids in your mouth.

But no need to worry, there is plenty of Vitamin D to go around. You can always get some Vitamin D from exposure form the sun. It is imperative that you know that only a few minutes of sun exposure is necessary otherwise you run the risk of incurring sunburn or skin cancer. There are tons of foods and beverages that have the right amount of Vitamin D. For instance fish like tuna, mackerel, salmon and trout have and adequate amount of Vitamin D which is great for maintain healthy teeth. Plus it is also present in fortified cereal, fortified diary, cod liver oil and beef liver.

Vitamin A

Vitamin A works wonders for your gums. Not having enough Vitamin A can be very bad for your gums. You see the tissue surrounding your guns and the mucous membrane there is protected by Vitamin A. It also aids in the healing of inflamed tissue.

There are tons of sources that include Vitamin A: liver, beef, eggs, milk and cheese. Start taking Vitamin A supplements too if you think that you are not getting this Vitamin enough form consuming whole foods. If you are taking Vitamin A just remember that Vitamin A is optimally absorbed when taken with fat so you have to take it when you are having a meal.

Vitamin B

When your body does not have enough B vitamins your gums start to recede and you may also experience toothache and oral sensitivity. Some common sources for B vitamins are fish, mushroom and meat.

Vitamin C

If you have loose teeth and bleeding gums it could be because of a Vitamin C deficiency. Like most other vitamins, Vitamin C not only improves your immune system but also shields you from infections that may damage your overall oral health.

When you are ensuring the proper levels of Vitamin C intake it is very simple to know which foods are high in it. Some foods such as citrus fruits and drinks have high quantities of Vitamin C.

Always remember to rinse your mouth after you have taken citrus so that the acid is balanced and it does not attack the tooth enamel. Other great sources of Vitamin C include cantaloupe, sprouts, Brussels, strawberries, green and red sweet peppers and kiwi. As with any nutrient or Vitamin that your body needs it is important that you get the daily recommended value of them naturally. You can take multivitamin tablets alongside these if you want.

Vitamins for Teens

For teens the right nutrition and vitamins are extremely important when it comes to their growth and development. This is the period where young girls face serious nutritional challenges and that will not only influence their development but their adult lives as well.

Unfortunately, the average teen will most probably skip breakfast, eat unhealthy cafeteria food and top it off with a fast food dinner. Therefore their bodies are not gaining any of the healthy Vitamins as recommended. The teenage years are a very unique period in life as it is a time of extreme physical and cognitive changes and experiences. It is important that those who do not get enough Vitamins from their daily food intake take supplements to meet the quota.

Plus, remember that each teenage girl is different and therefore it is important that their nutritional doses are addressed that fit each one's lifestyle. For instance some want to lose weight some want to gain muscle, and then there is the issue with menstruation, teenage pregnancy and some kids who have poor eating habits but are involved in a lot of physical activities.

Teenage girls need Vitamin A to boost their immune system, keep their eyes protected, heal skin and keep it healthy and most importantly facilitate cell growth. Food sources for these are liver, peaches, green leafy veggies, mangoes, eggs and milk.

Vitamin C is just as important as it promotes health and the immune system, It helps form collagen which is the tissue that helps hold cells together, it is imperative for maintaining healthy gums, teeth, blood vessels and bones, it aids in calcium absorption and iron that a teen consumes and the best part is that this Vitamin also contributes to brain function as well.

Vitamin C can be found in red berries, kiwi, grapefruit, oranges, guava, tomatoes, broccoli and red and green peppers.

Vitamin E protects the cells from damage and keeps the red blood cells in the body healthy. Teens can gain this Vitamin from foods like vegetable oils, leafy vegetables, avocado, nuts and whole grains.

DIY Vitamin Recipes for A Beautiful You

Citrus Face Cream - Topical Recipe

Ingredients

1 teaspoon powdered Vitamin B3

2 teaspoon Vitamin E oil

½ Oz vegetable glycerin

3 Oz Aloe Vera gel

1 teaspoon powdered L ascorbic acid

Grapefruit seed extract

Dark tinted glass container

Process

Start with stirring the powdered L ascorbic acid which is a form of Vitamin C. You can infuse that with your favourite homemade or store bought face cream. But if not then there is nothing wrong with starting from scratch. You can make your own cream by beating together the Aloe Vera gel, vegetable glycerin, Vitamin E oil and Vitamin B3. This is the recipe that makes basic face cream. You will need to add in a preservative as well. Go for the grape seed extract as it is natural and gentle on the skin.

Vitamin C Toner- Topical Recipe

Ingredients

1 teaspoon Vitamin C powder

1 Oz distilled water

Dark colored glass bottle

Process

Dissolve the Vitamin C powder in to the water. Put the mixture in fridge for around 14 days. Apply this topically to the skin after cleansing to help firm the skin and fight any inflammation or acne that you may be getting.

The Vitamin C Serum- Topical Recipe

Ingredients

¼ teaspoon Vitamin E

2 teaspoon glycerin

2 teaspoon distilled water

2 teaspoon Vitamin C powder

Process

Combine all the ingredients in a bowl until they are dissolved. Next, toss in the Vitamin E and glycerin. Put the entire mixture in a dark colour container. This is a basic serum that can be used at night time to help refine the pores.

Healing Face Cream- Topical Recipe

Ingredients

4 tablespoons coconut oil

6 drops lavender essential oil

2 teaspoon jojoba oil

12 Vitamin E oil capsules

½ cup Aloe Vera gel

Process

Mix slowly the coconut and jojoba oil along with the Aloe Vera gel. Put in the essential oils gently. After you let the cream rest for around 8 minutes you can place it in the fridge.

Hand Cream- Topical Recipe

Ingredients

12 tablespoons Vitamin E cream

12 tablespoons Vaseline

12 Oz baby lotion

Process

Simply mix all the ingredients with electric mixer and place in the jar. This is how most basic Vitamin E hand creams are made.

Taco Sauce - Food Recipe

Serves 4

Ingredients

Pinch of black pepper

Pinch of nutmeg

Pinch of cayenne pepper

½ teaspoon Dijon mustard

½ teaspoon salt

12 tablespoons firm tofu

2 cups almond milk (unsweetened)

8 tablespoons chopped carrots

10 Oz medium diced sweet potatoes

Process

Start by mixing sweet potatoes with milk and carrots. Turn the stove on medium heat and keep the food to simmer. Remember not to cover the food and wait til the veggies are tender, this will take around 18 minutes. Next in a separate bowl strain carrots and sweet potatoes, filtering out the almond milk. Measure the milk and if it mounts up to less than 1 ½ cup then add to it until it is that much.

Finally put all the ingredients in the blender and blend it until it is in smooth consistency.

Maple Salmon- Food Recipe

Serves 4

Ingredients

2 tablespoon maple syrup

4 salmon fillets (make sure they are at least an inch thick)

½ teaspoon roughly ground black pepper

2 teaspoon Dijon mustard

1 Oz Hoisin sauce

Process

Mix the mustard, sauce and syrup with the black pepper by whisking them. Put the salmon with its skin down in a broiler pan that is covered already with cooking spray. Coat the fish with the liquid mixture and broil to around 12 minutes.

Why Is It Good For You

Salmon contains Vitamin D, and some salmons have more of it than other types. For instance 3 ounces of Sockeye Salmon has 450 IU's of Vitamin D. It is marginally over the recommended dosage but it is nowhere near an unsafe amount.

Nuts Raisins and Carrots Salad- Food Recipe

Serves 2

Ingredients

1/8 cup cilantro leaves

½ Oz olive oil

Pinch of ground cayenne pepper

1/8 teaspoon ground cinnamon

¼ teaspoon paprika

¼ teaspoon crushed cumin

1 crushed garlic clove

1 ½ tablespoon freshly squeezed lemon juice

1/8 cup raisins

1 carrot, peeled and chopped into any shape you prefer

1/8 cup pistachios (shelled)

Salt and pepper

Process

Take a baking sheet and line it with pistachios. Put them in a p[reheated oven of 350 degrees and let them stay in there for 6 minutes. When you have taken them out and they have cooled chop them up into little tiny pieces.

Take a spare saucepan and boil some water with salt in it. Cook the carrots until they are crispy and tender. This would take around 6 minutes. Add raisins near the end and then rinse all the ingredients under cool water. Next take a medium bowl and beat together the cayenne, cinnamon, paprika, cumin, garlic and lemon juice together. You can top it with salt and pepper and mix it consistently. In the end add first oil. Use the pistachio, carrots and cilantro as the dressing. Toss before serving.

Why Is It Good For You?

Carrots have Vitamin A which is great for shielding us against cold and flu as well as help prevent cancer.

Apple and Sweet Potato Soup- Food Recipe

Serves 2

Ingredients

½ Oz mint, chopped

1/8 cup plain yogurt

½ tart Apple

1/8 teaspoon curry powder1/2 teaspoon honey

1 teaspoon white wine vinegar

2 cups veggie broth

2 small chopped garlic cloves

1 sliced jalapeno pepper

Salt and black pepper

½ an onion

½ Oz olive oil

1 ¾ pounds Sweet potato

Process

Start by placing sweet potatoes on a baking sheet and roasting them for an hour, in 400 degrees preheated oven. When the potatoes turn soft, wait until they cool down and then discard the skin after peeling it.

At the same time take a soup pot and heat the oil over medium heat. Start by adding the onion and salt and pepper, stir occasionally for around 15 minutes. Puree the soup in batches in a blender and then add that batch to a clean pot. Make sure the consistency is thick.

Next in a medium saucepan boil the honey, curry powder and vinegar to a boiling point and add apple. Stir the apple for a minute and then cut off the heat. When you serve add in some apple and yogurt in each serving with just a little bit of mint.

Why Is It Good For You?

The Vitamin A found in sweet potatoes is essential for maintaining healthy urinary, intestinal and respiratory tracts. Plus it works to keep the bacteria and viruses away from the body.

Egg Burrito- Food Recipe

Serves 4

Ingredient

4 tablespoons bottled salsa

8 tablespoons seeded and chopped tomato

4 fat free flour tortilla

8 tablespoons cheddar cheese, shredded

1 teaspoon butter

Cooking spray

½ teaspoon black pepper

¼ teaspoon kosher salt

2 teaspoon cilantro

1 Oz milk

4 eggs

Process

Beat together the eggs, cilantro, kosher salt, black pepper and milk together. Coat a non-stick skillet with a cooking spray and put the butter over medium flame. Now put in the egg mixture and stir.

Next sprinkle the cheese in the center of the tortilla, add the egg, tomato and salsa. Finally roll up the burrito. Do the same with the rest.

Why IS It Good For You?

To get Vitamin D from an egg it is important that you consume the egg yolk as well.

Healthy Greens- Food Recipe

Serves 4

Ingredients

¼ teaspoon red pepper flakes

½ pound spinach

4 garlic cloves

1 ½ tablespoon olive oil

¾ pounds greens

Process

Boil water with salt in it. Next put the greens into the water and blanch for around 2 minutes. Next put the greens on ice cold water, drain it, squeeze it dry and then set aside. At this point start garlic and oil in a pit over a medium low flame. Cook until the garlic is golden that takes around 8 to 10 minutes. Now take out the garlic from the pot and put it aside.

Turn up the heat and cook the greens for another 3 minutes. Put in the spinach and top it with red pepper flakes and salt. Cook until the spinach wilts and stir for a minute. Put the garlic back in the pot and start stirring.

Why Is It Great For You?

Swiss chard, sweet potatoes, apples, spinach, milk, mangoes, kale, eggs, collards, cheese, carrots , cantaloupe and apricots are fine sources of Vitamin A.

Grapefruit Brulee

Serves 3

Ingredients

½ cup Greek yogurt

¼ cup brown sugar

2 grapefruits

Process

Preheat the broiler and set the grapefruit (peeled) on the oven dish. Now sprinkle the fruit with brown sugar and broil until it is clear that the sugar has melted. You will know it has once the color turns darker. It will probably take around 5 minutes.

Serves

Ingredients

Process

Why is it great for you?

Vitamin in the Grapefruits has loads of energy. It has age and disease preventing benefits. To top it off it also has Vitamin A. It is recommended that you opt for a Vitamin C source like Grapefruits it is low in fat as well.

Frittata

Serves 8

Ingredients

30 ounces canned black beans

½ cup goat cheese

4 finely seeded and chopped jalapenos

2 cup cherry tomatoes cut in half

2 cups chopped onions

1 Oz olive oil

 1 teaspoon roughly ground pepper

1 teaspoon salt

4 omega 3 egg whites

12 omega 3 whole eggs.

Process

Start by heating the broiler over around 4 inches from the heat. In a dry bowl beat together the eggs, egg whites and add salt and pepper. Next in a non-stick oven proof skillet start heating the oil. You can add tomatoes and onions and cook these until they have completely softened. This takes around 6 minutes. You can combine the jalapeno peppers and egg mixture and continue by adding the goat cheese on top. Cover the skillet and cut down the heat to low. Give the eggs around 8 minutes to set.

You may place the frittata under the broiler and cook until you see it starting to brown. In a small saucepan you can cook beans until they are heated and add water if they seem too dry.

Serve wedges of the frittata with black beans.

Why Is It Great For You?

The Vitamin A which is found in this delicacy is great for improving weak eyesight and boosting your immune system.

Shrimp Kebabs with Jalapenos

Serves 2

Ingredients

1 plum pitted and cut into 6 sections

2 jalapenos

6 raw shrimp

¼ teaspoon salt

1` ½ tablespoon lime juice

½ teaspoon lime zest

½ Oz chopped cilantro

¾ Oz toasted sesame oil

Process

Start by whisking together the lime zest, cilantro, lime juice, salt and oil in a bowl. Set aside 2 tablespoons of this paste separately as you will need to use this as a dressing. You can reheat the gill to medium high. Continue by making 4 kebabs and alternating shrimp, plums, jalapenos and plums equally for two skewers. Grill this or about 8 minutes and serve with the reserved dressing.

Why is it great for you?

Shrimps are stuffed with Vitamin D, which you need for healthy skin and immune system. In this recipe you can even use peaches or nectarines in place of the plum.

Salmon

Serves 2

Ingredients

½ pound skinned salmon

¼ Oz Dijon mustard

1/8 teaspoon salt

½ garlic clove

15 sprigs mixed herbs

1 small lemon thinly sliced

Process

Begin by reheating the grill to medium high heat. You can lay 9 inch pieces of foil on a baking sheet, put the lemon slices in the middle of the foil and sprinkle the herbs over that. Mash and mix the garlic with salt so that it forms a paste. Continue by transferring it to a small dish and stirring in mustard and a bit of the reserved herbs. This combination will be coated in the fish. Next place the salmon on the foil. Cook the salmon in the grill until it look dark from the center. This takes around 18 minutes.

Why is it great for you?

Salmon is a great source for B Vitamins and Vitamin D.

Stuffed Pepper

Serves 8

Ingredients

½ cup raisins

2/3 cup chopped onion

1 cup rice

16 Oz ground beef

8 bell peppers

½ teaspoon ground cinnamon

2 teaspoon crushed cumin

1 Oz red wine vinegar

5o Oz of marinara sauce

Parsley (chopped) for garnishing

Process

Take a sizeable bowl and mix cinnamon, cumin, vinegar and sauce together. Slice off the top of each bell pepper, seed them carefully and reserve the tops. With your hand mix the rice, onions, sauce mixture, pepper, raisins and beef. Stuff this mixture into the peppers and put the stuffed peppers back on top.

Get a slow cooker and cook the peppers on low for 8 hours.

Why is it great for you?

Orange and yellow peppers are loaded with Vitamin C

Roasted Asparagus with Poached Eggs

Serves 2

Ingredients

1 ounce parmesan

2 eggs

¼ Oz cider vinegar

¼ Oz brown sugar

¼ cup balsamic vinegar

Salt

½ Oz olive oil

1 medium asparagus bunch

Process

Preheat your oven to 400 degrees. On a baking sheet put the asparagus with oil, sprinkle with salt. Bake this for 15 minutes. In a separate saucepan cook the balsamic vinegar and sugar over medium high heat until it is syrupy, then you can reduce it for another 5 minutes.

Simmer water up to two inches in a skillet over a medium flame. You can add cider vinegar and sprinkle with salt. You can break a single egg at a time into a cup and then tip this cup into the pan. You should simmer this until the whites are set and the yolks are soft but also slightly set, this takes around 3 minutes. Take a slotted spatula and scoop out the eggs individually and drain them on paper towels.

When serving top with the reduced balsamic and cheese with the egg on the side.

Why is it great for you?

The B vitamins in the asparagus are great for countering lethargy and can help prevent cold and flu.

Red Saffron Roast

Serves 4

Ingredients

1 tablespoon fresh mint chopped

Salt and pepper as required

¼ cup Nicoise olives

1 tablespoon sherry vinegar

Pinch of saffron

1/8 teaspoon red pepper flakes

¼ teaspoon paprika

1 chopped garlic clove

½ an onion

1 tablespoon olive oil

2 red bell peppers

Process

Start by broiling the peppers 4 inches from the heat. Turn them as their skin turns black. You want a mottled pattern. This will take about 20 minutes or so. Next you have to transfer everything into a bowl and cover the top with cling film. When they are cool enough to be handled you can easily take off their skins. Now cut each pepper lengthwise and slice them into wide strips.

Next you need to heat the oil in a large container over a medium flame. You can add onions and cook by stirring consistently. Now toss in the saffron, red pepper flakes, paprika and garlic. You need to cook this for an additional 2 minutes. Now add olives, vinegar and pepper. You can season them with salt and pepper and then cut the heat to low before you cook for an additional 3 minutes.

Why is it great for you?

The Vitamin C in these peppers is great for colds and is thought to be top multitasking vitamin.

Tuna with Sauce

Serves 2

Ingredients

½ tablespoon sunflower oil

½ pound yellow fin tuna (sushi grade), you can cut this in rectangular pieces.

½ tablespoon unhulled black sesame seeds

1 ½ tablespoon white sesame seeds

For the Sauce:

½ scallion sliced

1/8 teaspoon sesame oil

Pinch of red pepper flakes

4 teaspoons distilled white vinegar

1 teaspoon low sodium soy sauce

1 tablespoon orange juice

A little less than a ¼ cup carrot juice

1 teaspoon fresh ginger

1 teaspoon white miso

1 tablespoon mirin

Process

Start by making the Tuna. You have to mix the sesame seeds and then the tuna with it by pressing the meat into the seeds. Put the Tuna in a sauté pan over medium high flame. You need to cook the tuna until you see the white seeds going golden. After that all you need to do is place the tuna to a paper towel lined plate for a minute.

To make the sauce begin by mixing the sesame oil, red pepper flakes, vinegar, soy sauce, orange juice, carrot juice, ginger, miso and mirin. You only need to whisk this combination until the miso completely dissolves after with top it up with sliced scallion and you have yourself a dipping sauce.

Why is it great for you?

Tuna is one of the few sources of Vitamin D.

Spicy Avocado

Serves 4

Ingredients

4 whole wheat pita bread

2 sliced radishes

2 small cucumbers, peeled and diced

1 cup grape tomatoes cut in half

1 teaspoon salt and pepper

½ teaspoon crushed coriander

1 ½ teaspoon green Tabasco sauce

1 Oz orange juice

2 Avocados

Process

Stat by slicing the avocado's in half and removing the seed. Scoop out the avocado and then dice it into little chunky pieces. You can then put those in a bowl. Next toss in the coriander, Tabasco sauce and orange juice. Sprinkle some salt and pepper and mix.

Now add the radish, cucumber and tomatoes to this and serve equal portions with the pita bread.

Why is it great for you?

It has Vitamin E which is great for your skin.

Roasted Brussel Sprouts

Serves 2

Ingredients

¼ cup spicy kimchi

Salt and pepper as required

1 tablespoon olive oil

1 ounce of brussel sprouts with their ends trimmed and halved

Process

Take a baking sheet and align it with brussel sprouts with oil and salt and pepper. Put them in a 390°F preheated oven for around 20 minutes. Next add the kimchi to this mixture and cook until the kimchi is heated through. This only takes a couple of minutes.

Why is it great for you?

Brussel sprouts have a great amount of Vitamin K. This Vitamin is great for stopping bleeding wounds by enabling blood to clot. Plus the antioxidant helps boost the immune system.

Broccoli Soup

Serves 3

Ingredients

4 ounces light cheese

1/8 teaspoon black pepper

Less than a ¼ cup all-purpose flour

1 ¼ cup 2 % reduced fat milk

8 Ounce broccoli florets

1 ½ cup fat free chicken broth

1 ground garlic clove

½ cup onion finely diced

Cooking spray

Process

Start by heating a medium non-stick saucepan with cooking spray in it over a medium high flame. You can even add onion and garlic to this and sauté it for 2 minutes. Toss in the broccoli and the broth and boil this mixture over a medium high flame. When it starts boiling cut the flame to medium and cook for an additional 10 minutes.

Next mix the flour and the milk, stirring it until it is fully blended. You can then add the milk mixture to the broccoli mixture and then cook it for 5 minutes or until it is slightly thick. Mix in the pepper, cut the heat and stir in the cheese until it melts.

Why is it great for you?

It is a low calorie meal with a lot of Vitamin C.

Barley Salad

Serves 3

Ingredients

¼ cup barley

Less than a quarter cup of toasted sunflower seeds

½ of a large bunch of water cress, chopped into small pieces

1/8 cup minced fresh ill

¼ small red onion, finely chopped

½ cucumber diced

Ground pepper

¼ cup of extra virgin olive oil

½ teaspoon honey

1 teaspoon Dijon mustard

Less than a quarter cup fresh lemon juice

I carrot, diced

Salt as required

Process

Start by boiling around a quart of water in a pot and adding barley with a dash of salt in it. Continue by reducing it to a simmer and cooking uncovered until the barley is tender but chewy. Next drain the barley under cool water and place it in a bowl.

In a separate bowl whisk honey mustard, lemon juice and salt and pepper. Add this mixture and dill, red onion , cucumber and carrots to the bowl with barley. When you are serving, add the sunflower seeds and watercress to the salad and toss.

Why is it great for you?

Watercress has Vitamin K which develops bone density and strengthens them.

Vanilla Pudding

Serves 3

Ingredients

2 teaspoons butter

1 large egg yolk

1/8 cup half-and- half

Pinch of salt

1 ½ tablespoon cornstarch

1/3 cup sugar

Vanilla bean

1 1/34 cup milk (2% reduced fat)

Process

Start by taking a medium saucepan; Boil the vanilla bean and milk together into this. Also mix salt, cornstarch and sugar in a separate bowl. Stir them well. Stir the egg yolk mixture into the sugar mixture and eventually add half of the milk to the sugar mixture and stir constantly with a whisk. Put the milk mixture back into the pan and boil. Let it keep on cooking for a minute and do to stop stirring. Now remove the milk from the heat and add the butter, stir with a whisk until it completely dissolves the vanilla bean.

Pour the pudding into a bowl and wait for it to cool down. You can stir occasionally and then cover the top with a plastic wrap. Place it in the fridge.

Why is it great for you?

The egg yolks and milk are a great source of Vitamin D. Plus the pudding has very low sodium.

Tomato Salad Dressing

Makes 1 ½ cup

Ingredients

¼ cup olive oil

1/2 teaspoon paprika

1 chopped garlic clove

1 1/2 teaspoon light brown sugar

1 ½ Oz red wine vinegar

¾ pound tomatoes

Dash of salt and Pepper

Process

Cut an x shape with a knife on the bottom of the tomatoes. Bring the saucepan of water to a boil and add the tomatoes. You need to boil this for half a minute. Next, with a slotted spoon or a sieve take out the tomatoes and place them on a bowl. When they are cool enough to handle you can peel them. Put the peeled tomatoes in a blender. Add the paprika, garlic, sugar and vinegar and blend till you get a smooth consistency and while the mixture is being blended pour in the oil so that it gets mixed as it reaches the puree in a steady stream. Season the dressing with salt and pepper.

Why is it great for you?

The dressing is a great source of Vitamin E which prevents the production of harmful free radicals. The vitamin also helps respiratory health.

Hot Red Thai Curry with Veggies

Serves 2

Ingredients

½ lime

Less than a quarter of fresh cilantro

¼ teaspoon salt

1 teaspoon lime juice

½ tablespoon brown sugar

¼ pounds green beans

1 teaspoon red Thai curry paste

¼ cup vegetable broth

7 Ounce coconut milk

½ pound sweet potato

7 ounce extra firm tofu

2 teaspoons canola oil

Process

Start by taking a large non-stick skillet and heat oil in it on a medium high flame. Next add tofu and stir after two to three minutes until they start looking brown. Place all that in a plate. Next heat the remaining oil over medium high flame and toss in the sweet potato. Cook this for around 4 minutes and at this point add curry paste, broth and curry for flavor. Start boiling, and reduce to a simmer and cook. Make sure that you keep the pan covered. Also stir continuously.

Now toss in the tofu, green beans and brown sugar. You can return the food to simmer for another 4 minutes. Top it with cilantro and serve it with lime wedges.

Why is it great for you?

It may pack a lot of heat but it is a great source of Vitamin C.

Fish and Grape Pita

Serves 2

Ingredients

2 whole grain pita

Pic of crushed black pepper

4 teaspoon olive oil

2 tablespoon lemon juice

2 tablespoon fresh mint

1 Oz slivered almonds

1 cup halved red grapes

6 Ounces drained tuna

Process

Start by mixing the tuna, red grapes, almonds, mint black pepper and oil in a medium sized bowl and toss carefully. Serve them stiffed in the pita halves.

Why is it great for you?

Canned Tuna has long shelf life it is a source of Vitamin D. If you want a lot of Vitamin D then opt for the canned light tuna.

Sicilian Tuna

Serves 3

Ingredients

½ tablespoon mint

1/8 cup olive oil

4 ounce packed tuna

7 ½ ounce cannellini bean

Freshly ground kosher salt and pepper

1/8 cup thinly sliced red onion

1/2 garlic clove, crushed

1/8 cup Dijon mustard

¾ tablespoon red wine vinegar

1/8 cup olive oil

Process

Start by taking a small bowl and mixing red wine vinegar, minced garlic, Dijon mustard and the olive oil together. Use a whisk. Next toss in the red onion slices and let it cook for an additional 4 minutes. Sprinkle some salt and pepper on top.

In a sizeable bowl mix the beans and vinaigrette. Blend a third of this mixture in a processor until it is smooth. Next fold the mixture back into the beans and add tuna and olive oil. Mix in the beans, tuna and olive oil and then stir in two tablespoons of mint. Mix this until the tuna is not chunky anymore. Toast the bread until it is crispy and cut them in half. Next arrange the halves on a platter and put around two tablespoons of the bean mixture into each slice. Serve this with red onion and mint.

Why is it great for you?

It is super easy to make and comes with loads of Vitamin D.

Sesame Spinach

Serves 2

Ingredients

¾ Oz toasted sesame seeds

¾ tablespoon mirin

¾ tablespoon rice vinegar

¾ tablespoon naturally brewed soy sauce

¾ tablespoon sesame oil (toasted)

1 pound spinach

Process

Begin by preparing an ice water bath then set aside. Next boil water in a large pot and sprinkle over salt. Add spinach and cook it just until its wilted. This will take about 30 seconds. Drain the food and with your hands gently squeeze the excess water from it. Put the food on the work station and roughly chop the spinach and place it in a medium bowl before you set it aside.

In another small bowl mix together sesame oil, mirin, vinegar and soy sauce. Finally add the sesame seeds and the dressing to the spinach and mix.

Why is it great for you?

The spinach is full of carotenoids which helps protects against heart diseases.

Orange Chicken

Serves 2

Ingredients

¼ cup toasted slivered almonds

1 small cinnamon stick

1 tablespoon honey

¼ cup golden raisins

½ cup white wine

½ tablespoon canola oil

½ cup reduced chicken broth

2 boneless chicken breasts

1/8 teaspoon freshly ground pepper

¼ teaspoon salt

1 navel orange

Process

Take the juice of half of the orange and remove the zest. Reserve this. Take a bowl and mix salt pepper and flour in it. Coat the chicken with this flour and then put the broth in the leftover flour. Whisk to mix completely. Next heat the oil in a non-stick skillet over a medium flame. Cook the chicken until it is browned. It will take around 3 to 4 minutes on each side. Transfer this to a plate.

Take a pan and pour wine in it, cook the wine for a minute and then add the flour and broth mixture to it. In the flour broth mixture add the orange juice and the zest, cinnamon sticks, honey, raisins and a pinch of salt. Boil this. Make sure that you cut down the heat to a simmer and then out the chicken in the pan to cook along with the juice. Take around 12 minutes. Next take out the cinnamon sticks and serve in a plate with the sauce over the chicken and the range slices on the side.

Why is it great for you?

The savory ingredients pack a lot of beneficial Vitamin C.

Chicken Tender Wrap

Serves 2

Ingredients

2 tortillas

½ cup cucumber chopped

1 small tomato chunks

½ pound chicken tenders

1/8 teaspoon freshly ground pepper

1/8 teaspoon salt

1 teaspoon garlic chopped

1 ½ tablespoon garlic crushed

1 ½ tablespoon olive oil

1/8 cup lemon juice

¼ cup fresh mint

½ cup fresh parsley

Less than a quarter cup whole wheat couscous

¼ cup water

Process

Begin by boiling the water in a saucepan. Mix in the couscous and cut off the heat. Cover the pan and let it cook for 5 minutes. Set this aside. Take a medium sized bowl and mix together the garlic, oil, lemon juice, pinch of salt and pepper, mint and parsley. In a separate bowl add the chicken tenders and half a tablespoon of the parsley combination with the remaining salt. Place these tenders in a skillet and cook through on a medium flame. Remove them from the heat and cut them into bite sized pieces.

The reaming parsley mixture that you have, stir it into the couscous with the tomato and the cucumber.

Divide the couscous mixture and the tenders into each tortilla. Roll the wraps like a burrito and serve.

Why is it great for you?

The meal is packed with Vitamin C and a healthy dose of herbs.

Berry Yogurt

Serves 2

Ingredients

2 teaspoons finely chopped pistachios

½ cup greek yogurt

¼ cup heavy cream

Squirt of lime juice

Less than a quarter cup of honey

¼ pint blueberries

Process

In a blender blend the blueberries, juice, lime and honey. Press the mixture through a mesh sieve and take out the seeds and the skin. Discard these. Place this in a container and cover it with a plastic wrap. Next refrigerate until it is cold for about ten minutes.

With an electric mixer and a whisk whip the cream until the peaks are stiff in consistency and then combine the cream into the yogurt.

With your hands gently mix the blueberry blend into the yogurt mixture. Spoon them into glasses and chill.

Pork with Blueberry Puree

Serves 2

Ingredients

1 bunch watercress

1 tablespoon olive oil

1 ½ teaspoon Dijon mustard

½ pork tenderloin

2 teaspoon red wine vinegar

Ground salt and pepper as required

½ minced shallot

½ tablespoon crushed ginger

½ cups seedless red grapes

1 cup blueberries, frozen

Process

Start by heating the broiler with rack set 4 inches from the heat. Now in a small saucepan mix the shallots, salt, pepper, water, blueberry, grapes and ginger in a saucepan. Boil it over a high flame. Cut the heat to a medium high flame and cook until the grapes break apart and the mixture gets thick. After that pour in the vinegar.

While the chutney

Why is it great for you?

Pork is a source of B Vitamins.

Strawberry Shortcake

Serves 5

Ingredients

1 cup frozen fat free topping (whipped)

¾ teaspoon granulated sugar

1 of an egg white, whisked lightly

Cooking spray

¼ teaspoon vanilla extract

1/3 cup buttermilk

3 tablespoons chilled butter

¼ teaspoon baking soda

¼ teaspoon salt

½ teaspoon grated lemon rind

1 teaspoon baking powder

1/4 cup sugar

1 cup al purpose flour

Shortcake

2 cups sliced strawberries

Process

Begin by preparing the strawberries. Start by mixing the strawberries and half of the sugar together and set them aside keeping them covered.

Next preheat the oven to 400 degrees and while its on start working on the shortcake. Mix the four with the baking soda in a large bowl. Toss in the butter and mix it well (you can use a pastry blender here). Next combine the vanilla and buttermilk separately and mix them in with the flour as well.

The dough will be sticky now so put it on a flour-covered surface and knead with hands. The dough will not be that big so shape it into a circle and lay it on top of a baking sheet coated in cooking spray. Do not forget to brush the top with egg white and sprinkle with ¾ teaspoons of sugar. Put the tray in the oven and bake for around 13 to 15 minutes.

Once the shortcake is cool enough to handle. Split in half horizontally with a knife and let the two layers cool separately too.

Tale a plate and place the bottom half of the shortcake on it. Spread the whipped topping over this and evenly arrange the strawberries over this. Now cover it with the second shortcake layer.

Why is it great for you?

One cup of strawberries has 85 mg of Vitamin C and to top it has very low calories.

Kiwi Umbrella

Serves 3

Ingredients

4 cups canned pineapples with juice

1 ½ tablespoon cream of coconut

1/8 cup Midori

1/8 cup light rum

1 ½ cup ice

2 kiwifruit (peeled and divided)

Process

Blend 2 kiwifruits in a blender. Put the remaining kiwi aside. Add the rest of the ingredients including the ice in the blender and blend until it reaches a smooth consistency. When you take out the beverage run it though a sieve and divide it evenly among 3 glasses.

Why is it great for you?

A single kiwi has 70 mg of Vitamin C.

Chicken and Cheese Bell Peppers

Serves 2

Ingredients

1 ½ ounce fontina cheese

2 teaspoons low fat mayonnaise

6 ounce loaf rosemary focaccia

Pinch of salt and pepper

½ tablespoon red wine vinegar

3 ½ ounce red bell peppers (bottle roasted)

1/8 teaspoon salt

1/8 teaspoon crushed red pepper

1/3 teaspoon ground fennel seeds

½ teaspoon sugar

½ cup vertically sliced onion

Cooking spray

3 crushed garlic cloves

1/8 teaspoon dried thyme

1/8 teaspoon dried marjoram

1 teaspoon olive oil

½ tablespoon Dijon mustard

½ tablespoon lemon juice

½ pound chicken breast halves

Process

Begin by placing the chicken between two sheets of plastic wrap. Pound the chicken with a mallet or a rolling pin until it is only ¾ of an inch thick. Now mix juice, thyme, marjoram, oil, mustard, chicken and 1 garlic clove in a zip lock bag and marinate by refrigerating it for two hours.

At this point take a sizeable non-stick skillet and put it on medium high heat. Put cooking spray on the pan and sauté the remaining garlic cloves, crushed red pepper, fennel, sugar, onion and garlic cloves for a minute.

Next add roasted bell peppers and cook for around 4 minutes. After that mix in the black pepper and vinegar. Take the chicken out of the zip lock bag and grill it on a medium high flame. Grill for 5 minutes on each side and cool slightly then cut the chicken into slices. Next spread the cut sides of the bread with mayonnaise and put cheese on the bottom of eh bread. Now evenly arrange the pepper and chicken mixture over cheese. Cover it with the other half of the bread. Put this on the grill for around 3 minutes on each side.

Cut this load into quarters before serving.

Why is it great for you?

This delicious meal is not only full of mouth-watering ingredients but is packed with Vitamin C.

Lamb and Papaya

Serves 3

Ingredients

½ teaspoon chopped jalapeno pepper

½ tablespoon lemon juice

1/8 cup cilantro

¼ cup chopped red onion

½ cup papaya (peeled and diced)

6 lamb loin chops

1/8 teaspoon black pepper

¼ teaspoon salt

1 teaspoon garam masala

Process

Before you handle the ingredients preheat the broiler. Mix the salt, pepper and garam masala and then coiat this blend on the lamb chops. Arrange the lamb in one layer on the broiler pan and broil for 4 minutes on every side. take them off the heat and then sprinkle with 1/8 teaspoon of salt.

Separately mix the papaya and the rest of the ingredients and stir. Serve this with the lamb.

Why is it great for you?

Vitamin C is stacked in papayas. Each has 188mg of this vitamin.

The Nutritious Chocolate Milkshake

Serves 4

Ingredients

1 Oz agave syrup

2 tablespoon cocoa powder

2 cups 1% low fat milk

1 cup low fat chocolate frozen yogurt (Vitamin D fortified)

Process

Put all the ingredients in the blender and blend until they are all smooth. Divide the shake equally among 4 glasses and serve.

Why is it great for you?

The recipe gives you a good dose of calcium and 50 IU of Vitamin D per serving. If you want you can use an alternative of the frozen yogurt that is the Vitamin D fortified soy milk.

Pasta with Beans

Serves 4

Ingredients

4 tablespoons pecorino romano cheese

Freshly ground pepper as required

½ cup sliced basil

4 tablespoons black olives

4 ripe tomatoes

2 large ground garlic cloves

30 ounce cannellini beans

2 tablespoon olive oil

8 ounces whole wheat pasta shells

Process

Start by taking a sizeable saucepan and boiling water in it. Toss in the pasta and wait until they are tender. About 10 minutes then drain.

Take a sizeable skillet and over a medium flame put the oil, garlic and beans for 3 to 5 minutes. Cut off the heat and toss in the tomatoes, basil, olives and pepper. Stir a bit and serve the paste with the bean mixture and cheese on the top.

Why is it great for you?

The recipe is stacked with your daily dose of Vitamin C.

Pumpkin Seed and Quinoa Salad

Serves 2

Ingredients

1/8 cup toasted pumpkin seeds

2 lime wedges

½ ripe avocado sliced

1 ripe, medium tomato cut into wedges

½ of a head red leaf lettuce

1/8 cup chopped cilantro leaves

½ of a jalapeno pepper, diced and seeded

½ of a red pepper, diced and seeded

1 corn ear kernels

¾ cups quinoa

Sea salt

¼ cup olive oil

½ garlic clove ground

½ teaspoon chili powder

½ teaspoon cumin, crushed

Process

Start by boiling water in a small saucepan and stirring in the quinoa with salt. Put it back on boil and et it simmer with the lid on. This will take around 15 minutes. Next turn off the heat and toss in the kernels on top of the quinoa. Let this cook for an additional 5 minutes. Stir the corn into the quinoa and take it off the pan and then spread it on a baking sheet for about 20 minutes.

In a separate bowl mix the salt, oil, garlic, chili powder, cumin and lemon juice. Put the quinoa, cilantro, jalapeno, scallions, cucumber, red pepper and corn. Add ¼ cup of the dressing and salt to taste.

Place lettuce leaves on a serving platter and place the quinoa salad in the middle. Now put the avocado, tomato and lime over the leaves and serve.

Why is it great for you?

Corn and Avocados are great sources Of the B Vitamins which include folate which is particularly good for pregnant women.

Herb and Mushroom Soup

Serves 4

Ingredients

1/8 cup dry sherry

¼ cup half and half

½ cup 1% low fat milk

2 cups fat free chicken broth

4 ounce button mushrooms, sliced

3 cups mushroom shitake caps (sliced)

1/8 teaspoon freshly ground black pepper

1/8 teaspoon salt

1 teaspoon chopped thyme

1 teaspoon garlic

¾ cups chopped onion

1 teaspoon butter

½ cup dried porcini mushrooms

½ cup boiling water

1 tablespoon all-purpose flour

Process

Put the flour in a skillet over medium high flame and cook for 2 minutes. Then transfer the flour to a small plate and let it cool

Next mix the mushrooms and boiling water in a bowl and put the lid on it and let it steep for 20 minutes. Use a sieve to strain the porcini mushrooms but do not discard the liquid, and chop the mushrooms.

Now melt the butter in an oven over a medium high flame and toss in the onion. Sauté the food for 5 minutes or until it is tender. Add in the thyme, garlic, salt and pepper and sauté it for half a minute. Stir in the shitake mushrooms and cook for 3 minutes. Finally add the porcini mushrooms and broth to pan.

Next mix the saved porcini's liquid to the toasted flour and beat the ingredients with a whisk. Put this combination in the pan and wait till it boils, even it does lower the heat to a simmer for only 15 minutes without the lid.

Now stir in the milk and let it simmer for an additional 10 minutes. Remove the stove from the heat and pour in the sherry and half and half. Next put the soup in the blender and blend it until it is smooth. Return this to the pan and then warm the soup thoroughly and serve after sprinkling parsley.

Why is it great for you?

The mushrooms in this soup are one of the few sources of Vitamin D and this is because these mushrooms have been exposed to Ultraviolet rays. The recipe gives 325 IUs of Vitamin D in each serving.

Avocado, Cheese and Tortilla Soup

Serves 4

Ingredients

3 lime wedges

1/3 Mexican melting cheese, shredded

1 cup tortilla chips, broken

½ ripe avocado cut into cubic pieces

¼ teaspoon salt

2 cups chopped chard

7 ounce extra firm tofu

½ sprig epazote

2 cups water

2 cups vegetable broth

1 ½ garlic clove

1 medium white onion

4 teaspoons extra virgin olive oil

7 ½ ounce fire roasted diced canned tomatoes

1 ½ large dried pasilla

Process

Start by toasting the chilies over an open flame with metal tongs. Once cool enough to handle seed the chilies and toss them on the blender with tomatoes and the canned juice. Do not completely puree them. Next heat 2 tablespoons of oil in an oven and add onion and garlic and cook stirring until they are golden. Scoop up the onion and garlic with a slotted spoon and transfer the blender with the tomato mixture until its smooth.

Cut the heat on the pot to medium and its hot add the puree and stir constantly until it's thickened to the consistency of tomato paste. Add the broth and water and boil then adjust the heat to a simmer.

At this point you need to drain the tofu and pat dry and then cut into small cubic pieces. Cook the tofu in a pan over medium heat. Toss in the tofu and then cook in a single layer where you have to stir every couple of minutes until the food gets brown. Now add this to the soup and let it simmer for around half an hour.

In the end put chard in the soup, sprinkle some salt cook for a few more minutes.

Why is it great for you?

The soup has delicious earthy flavors and is packed with Vitamin C.

Chili Casserole

Serves 4

Ingredients

For the chili:

1/8 teaspoon cayenne pepper

½ teaspoon sweet paprika

½ tablespoon crushed cumin

1 ½ tablespoon chili powder

14 ounce can tomatoes

7 ½ ounce kidney beans

½ pound lean ground beef

1 ½ minced garlic cloves

½ chopped green bell pepper,

½ of an onion finely chopped

½ tablespoon canola oil

For the cornbread:

¾ cups extra sharp cheddar cheese

¼ cup cilantro

1 tablespoon canola oil

¾ cups low fat milk

1 egg, lightly whisked

Pinch of salt

¼ teaspoon baking soda

½ teaspoon baking powder

1 tablespoon sugar

1/3 cup whole wheat flour

¾ cups cornmeal

Process

Start with the chili. Heat the oil on medium heat in the oven and add onion until it begins to soften. This will take around 3 minutes only. Add the bell pepper and the garlic and then cook for a minute. After that add beef and cook breaking it up with a wooden spoon until they are browned this will only take a couple of minutes. Next stir in the beans, tomatoes and the juice along with cayenne, paprika, chili powder and cumin. Boil all these ingredients and once it does cut the heat to a simmer and cook for 20 minutes.

Preheat the oven to 350 degrees Fahrenheit and coat a baking dish with cooking spray.

Now when you start preparing the cornbread beat together the cornmeal, flour, sugar, baking soda, salt and baking powder in a sizeable bowl. After this add the wet ingredients to the dry ingredients including cilantro and stir until it has just combined.

Put the chili on the baking dish and top it with the shredded cheese. Now gently spread the cornbread batter over this and back this or around 20 minutes. You will know it is ready once the top pops back.

Why is it great for you?

The ingredients list may not be brief but it is very easy to cook and filled with nutritious Vitamin C.

Bacon Pasta

Serves 3

Ingredients

¼ cup sliced scallions for garnish

Less than a quarter cup reduced fat sour cream

14 ounce crushed tomatoes

½ tablespoon all-purpose flour

¼ tablespoon freshly ground pepper

2 teaspoons Cajun seasoning

1 ½ garlic cloves

½ bell pepper, cut into slices

½ pound boneless chicken breast

½ sweet onion, sliced

2 teaspoons canola oil

4 ounce whole wheat rotini or fusilli

Process

Boil water in a large pot and cook the pasta until it is tender, this will take around 10 minutes. Drain it.

Add bacon, onion and oil in the oven and cook over medium heat. Stir occasionally until the food begins to brown this will take 2 minutes. Next add the chicken, garlic, bell pepper, pepper and Cajun seasoning. Cook for about 4 minutes.

Add flour and stir. After that put in tomatoes and their juice and bring everything to a simmer. Cook until the sauce thickens and the chicken is cooked through. This will only take 2 minutes. Combine the pasta into the sauce and top it with scallions.

Why is it great for you?

The zesty taste of the pasta is mouthwatering and is a great source of Vitamin C.

Orange Cocktail

Serves 2

Ingredients

2 ounces blood orange juice

2 ounces citrus vodka

Process

Take an ice filled shaker and mix the two ingredients in the shaker. Strain the liquid into a chilled martini glass.

Why is it great for you?

You can get some of your share of Vitamin D from this cocktail beverage. It's better if you use fortified orange juice. You can also switch the vodka with citrus flavored sparkling water.

Spinach and Autumn Greens

Serves 4

Ingredients

¼ teaspoon red pepper flakes

½ pound spinach

4 sliced garlic cloves

1 ½ tablespoon olive oil

¾ pounds autumn greens, washed and sliced

Process

Start by boiling a big pot of salted water. Put the greens into the water and let them be for 4 minutes. Next transfer the greens in a bowl of ice cold water. Drain and dry them.

Take a large skillet and heat the oil and garlic until the garlic is golden around the edges. This will take around 6 to 7 minutes. Take out the garlic from the skillet and reserve. Raise the heat and toss in the greens and cook these for an additional 3 minutes. Toss in the spinach with pepper flakes and salt. Cook all this until the spinach wilts. Put the garlic back into the pan and stir.

Why is it great for you?

This healthy recipe is a great source of Vitamin A.

Yogurt and Shrimp Pasta

Serves 8

Ingredients

½ cup toasted pine nuts

1 teaspoon ground pepper

2 tablespoon extra virgin olive oil

6 tablespoons lemon juice

½ cup flat leaf parsley

3 cups low fat yogurt

¾ teaspoon kosher salt

2 minced small garlic cloves

2 cups green peas

2 big red bell peppers

2 bunch asparagus. Sliced

24 ounces peeled and deveined raw shrimp

12 ounces whole wheat spaghetti

Process

Start by boiling the spaghetti in a large pot only two minutes earlier than what the package instructs. Add the peas, bell peppers, asparagus and shrimp to this. Drain this.

Grind the garlic and salt until it forms into a paste and min in pepper, oil, lemon juice, parsley and yogurt. Top it with pine nuts before serving.

Why is it great for you?

You have a garlicky Middle Eastern inspired yogurt sauce that is not only tempting but is filled with Vitamin C.

Sea Scallops Salad

Serves 8

Ingredients

For the salad:

2 tablespoons canola oil

2 pounds sea scallops

½ teaspoon ground pepper

½ teaspoon kosher salt

4 teaspoons coriander seeds

4 tangerines

12 cups torn frisee

12 cups baby spinach

For the vinaigrette:

½ teaspoon ground pepper

½ teaspoon salt

2 teaspoon Dijon mustard

4 teaspoon chopped spring herbs

2 tablespoon spring herbs

2 tablespoon shallot, minced

8 teaspoons white wine vinegar

4 tablespoons tangerine

1 teaspoon tangerine

4 tablespoons olive oil

Process

Start by preparing the vinaigrette. Take a medium bowl and whisk together the salt, pepper, mustard, herbs, shallot, vinegar, tangerine zest and juice and olive oil. To prepare the salad combine the frisee, spinach and tangerine fragments.

Roughly chop the coriander seeds and mix the kosher salt and pepper in a separate bowl. Coat this on both scallops' sides. Take a large non-stick skillet over medium high heat until. Toss in the scallops and cook until they get a golden brown crust and are cooked through, you will know this once you see that they are entirely opaque. This means around 3 minutes on each side.

Serve the salad with scallops on top.

Why is it great for you?

This is a Vitamin C rich and easy to make dinner salad.

Eggplants, Peanuts and Chilli

Serves 8

Ingredients

½ cup chopped fresh cilantro

½ cup roasted cashews or peanuts

4 large ripe mangoes, peeled and cut into cubic pieces

8 cups torn romaine lettuce

4 bunches scallions

3 cups cooked lentils

½ teaspoon freshly ground pepper

½ teaspoon salt

½ cup honey

½ cup prepared salsa

2/3 cup lime juice

4 medium eggplants

5 teaspoons curry powder

5 teaspoons chili powder

8 tablespoons olive oil

Process

Begin by preheating the oven to 500 degrees. Mix 2 tablespoons of oil with 4 teaspoon of chili powder and 4 teaspoons of curry powder in a bowl. Add eggplant into this and toss. Spread the eggplant on a baking sheet and roast for around 20 minutes.

Next thoroughly mix the remaining 6 tablespoons of oil and the remaining chili and curry powder along with salt, pepper, honey, salsa and 2/3 cups lime juice.

Why is it great for you?

This delicious recipe is filed with a healthy dose of Vitamin C.

Cherry and Bulgur Salads

Serves 8

Ingredients

½ cup chopped walnuts

1 cup fresh herbs

1 pound pitted fresh cherries

2 minced shallots

6 tablespoons lemon juice

4 tablespoons walnut oil

Salt and pepper required

2 cups bulgur wheat

Process

In a medium saucepan boil water with the lid on and then add ½ teaspoon salt and bulgur and mix to combine. Lower the heat and cook until the water is entirely absorbed and the bulgur is tender.

Next in a medium bowl mix the shallot, lemon juice and oil together and sprinkle it with salt and pepper. Add bulgur to this and then toss to mix. Refrigerate this without covering it for 10 to 15 minutes.

When serving add walnuts, herbs and cherries to the bulgur mixture and toss this to mix. Sprinkle it with salt and pepper.

Why is it great for you?

Great source of Vitamin C

Beauty and Health Go Hand In Hand

For Strong Nails

Studies show that biotin supplements actually help in strengthening brittle nails. Biotin is also known as Vitamin H and is one of the B complex Vitamins which work to aid your body to metabolize proteins and fats. Dermatologists recommend a daily 5 milligram supplement of each of these.

Zap Those Blemishes

Oral probiotics are great in helping combat acne and cut down on inflammation and oxidative stress which if you do not know is the internal damage that is done by free radicals. A recent report analysed and found that gut microbes in the gastrointestinal tract are a major source for acne. Therefore it is important to know that what is going on in your intestines shows on your skin. Things like alcohol, stress, too much sugar and some birth control pills can all contribute to having acne-prone skin.

For an Awesome Mood

For a better mood omega 3 fatty acids have the solution as they are known to elevate your mood. A Canadian study showed that adults with major depression who took fish oil supplements for eight weeks faced a major improvement in their mood compared to the adults who took a placebo.

For relieving Stress

High intakes of Vitamin C help relieve stress. One study found that participants who took 3000mg every day experienced lower blood pressure and stress as compared to the subjects who only took a placebo. What happens is that Vitamin C ruins the effect of cortisol, which is a stress hormone released by the adrenal glands. The recommended dose is 75 mg. However it would be much wiser if you talk to your nutritionist before you start taking the Vitamin.

For Great Eyesight

The B complex Vitamins are known to keep your eyesight strong. A recent study found that women who take B complex Vitamins continuously have lesser chances of macular degeneration which is a retina disease that leads to blurred vision and even blindness.

A Clear Head

Vitamin D works great for a clear head and memory improvement. Low levels of Vitamin D affects brain functioning in women.

How to go Supplement Shopping

If the supplement aisle at the store overwhelms, you it is perfectly normal. There are just so many different brands claiming so many things. Let's keep in mind that the supplement business industry is making billions and that is also mostly because unlike other meds supplements do not necessarily have to go through clinical testing before they are ready to be sold in the market. This also means that not all labels actually do what they claim.

The best part is that you do not have to spend a whole lot of cash in order to get high quality supplements; you just have to be a smart shopper.

The first thing that you need to do is research. Websites review sites can be reliable. Look for what supplement or brand you are interested in.

A quality seal means that a supplement has undergone independent testing and that it really is what it claims.

Whole food supplements are the supplements that try to copy the effect of real food when consumed. The difference is that supplements are more concentrated and only provide a specific Vitamin.

How to Store Vitamins Properly?

It does make a huge difference where you store the Vitamins that you take. It could be the kitchen, the bathroom, the counter or the refrigerator.

Not the Fridge

When you read the instructions on a bottle and it says that you must store the pills in a cool and dry place it does not mean that you should store your supplements in the fridge. The fridge is definitely cool but it is also has a lot of moisture. Moistures cuts down on Vitamin shelf life and render it useless. The only supplements that can be inside the refrigerator are the ones with specific directions on the packing about refrigeration storage.

Not the Bathroom

The classic place for storing all medicine and supplements is the medicine cabinet. By storing the vitamins in the same room as you take a bath and shower means that you are exposing them to moisture coupled with heat on a daily basis; this combination rapidly deteriorates the effectiveness of any medications stored there.

Not the Kitchen

Since all Vitamins are taken alongside meals it makes sense that you would want to store them near where you keep your food. You cannot store them in the kitchen as the temperature in the kitchen rises and falls all the time. Instead choose to store them in the dining room or the nook where you have breakfast. If you have a place that is away from direct heating and cooling place such as stoves ovens and fridges then you can keep them there.

Nutritional supplements may seem that they are natural but they are also potentially toxic if you consume them in very high doses. It is time that you stopped the habit of taking them out of their original packaging. Avoid cabinets that are close to windows or pipes. This way you are storing them in a dry place and out of reach of children.

A reason that you should store your Vitamins in the original containers is because some of them require special packaging to retain the optimal potency and the supplements that come in dark tinted bottles are the ones that are most likely to lose their effectiveness when exposed to light. All of us do things that are most convenient for us, like putting the vitamins from smaller to larger containers and combining all the supplements that you are supposed to take in a day in one container so that things are convenient.

Always remember that Vitamins lose their effectiveness with age. So you better check for the expiration date before you buy the supplements. Consuming expired supplements are not nor toxic but they are not effective either. Therefore, always remember to check for the expiration date before you buy the supplements.

Know Your Vitamins Next Time You Are Makeup Shopping

For many years Vitamins have been treated as highly valuable ingredients in all kinds of cosmetics. They give the skin loads of benefits, some of which are suppression of pigmentation and bruises, refinement of the skin and stimulation of collagen synthesis. Then there are the antioxidants and anti-inflammatory effects. The antioxidant effect is favored since free radicals created by UV light or pollutants are neutralized and cannot damage skin cells anymore. Vitamins can then significantly improve the effects of cosmetics.

Provitamin B5 and Vitamin A, C and E are the ones that are mostly used in cosmetics.

Provitamin B5

Provitamin B5 or what it is commonly known in the cosmetic industry, D Panthenol has been used in hair care products for a very long time now. It increases hair volume (by raising the water content) and makes dry and stiff hair more elastic.

D Panthenol is inactive but is easily converted into pantothenic acid in the skin. Pantothenic acid is then used as a vital part in the skin cell's energy cycle. Panthenol also pulls water to the upper layers of the skin and because of that it is a great softener and moisturizer. Panthenol also encourages epithelization of the skin. This means that the skin can heal and rejuvenate quickly, letting young-looking skin show through.

Vitamin C

Vitamin C is a popular cosmetic ingredient that due to its ability to quench UV induced free radicals and to regenerate Vitamin E which is a potent antioxidant. There are 3 forms most commonly used in cosmetics; these are the L ascorbic acid, ascorbyl palmitate and magnesium ascorbyl.

Ascorbyl palmitate is a soluble form of Vitamin C. Its best feature is that it is stable when it is incorporated in cosmetic formulas and has a neutral pH.

L -ascorbic acid is water soluble and must be formulated at low pH in order to stay active. In many clinical trials Vitamin C has acts as an anti-inflammatory and an antioxidant agent. When it is applied on UV burns, Vitamin C lowers redness in half of the time quicker than it would otherwise take. And that is not the end of it either. Eczema and psoriasis also heal quickly once treated with Vitamin C.

Moreover Vitamin C does more than that, it is supposed to boost collagen synthesis which is why it is also dubbed as an anti-ageing element.

Vitamin A

The primary reason that Vitamin A is used in cosmetics is because it is able to stabilize keratinization - a condition which makes the skin look rough. Vitamin A works to control the growth of the skin cells and lowers roughness and skin wrinkling. This is also why it's called the skin normalizing and rejuvenating agent.

In cosmetics Vitamin A is in the form of retinol (vitamin A alcohol), retinyl palmitate (Vitamin A esters), retinal (Vitamin A aldehyde) and a trans-retinoic acid (tretinoin).

Vitamin E

Vitamin E is known to prevent free radicals from harming us. It also works to cut down on UV induced erythema, sunburn, edema and lipid peroxidation.

Vitamin E has also been recorded to remove signs of aging and wrinkles. It is thought that this is due to the excellent moisturizing properties of the Vitamin.

References

AB, Nobel Media, "Sir Frederick Hopkins - Nobel Lecture: The Earlier History of Vitamin Research" http://www.nobelprize.org/nobel_prizes/medicine/laureates/1929/hopkins-lecture.html (accessed 11 Dec 2014).

Acar, U., H. I. Atilgan, D. E. Acar, Z. Yalniz-Akkaya, N. Yumusak, M. Korkmaz, and G. Koca. "The Effect of Short-Term Vitamin E against Radioiodine-Induced Early Lacrimal Gland Damage." *Ann Nucl Med* 27, no. 10 (2013): 886-91.

All About Vitamins and Minerals : Key Nutrients for Optimum Health. No Nonsense Health Guide. Stamford, CT: Longmeadow Press, 1989.

Almadan, M. S., B. H. al Awamy, and I. A. al Mulhim. "Nutritional Vitamin B12 Deficiency in Infancy." *Indian J Pediatr* 60, no. 5 (1993): 683-5.

Amann, P. M., C. Luo, R. W. Owen, C. Hofmann, M. Freudenberger, D. Schadendorf, S. B. Eichmuller, and A. V. Bazhin. "Vitamin a Metabolism in Benign and Malignant Melanocytic Skin Cells: Importance of Lecithin/Retinol Acyltransferase and Rpe65." *J Cell Physiol* 227, no. 2 (2012): 718-28.

Amini, M., M. Khosravi, H. R. Baradaran, and R. Atlasi. "Vitamin B12 Supplementation in End Stage Renal Diseases: A Systematic Review." *Med J Islam Repub Iran* 29, (2015): 167.

Andrieux, P., P. Fontannaz, T. Kilinc, and E. C. Gimenez. "Pantothenic Acid (Vitamin B5) in Fortified Foods: Comparison of a Novel Ultra-Performance Liquid Chromatography-Tandem Mass Spectrometry Method and a Microbiological Assay (Aoac Official Method 992.07)." *J AOAC Int* 95, no. 1 (2012): 143-8.

Antille, C., C. Tran, O. Sorg, P. Carraux, L. Didierjean, and J. H. Saurat. "Vitamin a Exerts a Photoprotective Action in Skin by Absorbing Ultraviolet B Radiation." *J Invest Dermatol* 121, no. 5 (2003): 1163-7.

Baggerly, L. L. "Vitamin D: Dosages to Optimize Serum Levels." *Altern Ther Health Med* 21, no. 3 (2015): 14-15.

Barnett, M. L., and G. Szabo. "Effect of Vitamin a on Epithelial Morphogenesis in Vitro." *Exp Cell Res* 76, no. 1 (1973): 118-26.

Beck, M. A. "Increased Virulence of Coxsackievirus B3 in Mice Due to Vitamin E or Selenium Deficiency." *J Nutr* 127, no. 5 Suppl (1997): 966S-970S.

Bikle, D. "Vitamin D: Production, Metabolism, and Mechanisms of Action." In *Endotext*, edited by L. J. De Groot, P. Beck-Peccoz, G. Chrousos, K. Dungan, A. Grossman, J. M. Hershman, C. Koch, R. McLachlan, M. New, R. Rebar, F. Singer, A. Vinik and M. O. Weickert. South Dartmouth (MA), 2000.

Bito, T., Y. Matsunaga, Y. Yabuta, T. Kawano, and F. Watanabe. "Vitamin B12 Deficiency in Caenorhabditis Elegans Results in Loss of Fertility, Extended Life Cycle, and Reduced Lifespan." *FEBS Open Bio* 3, (2013): 112-7.

Blatt, D. H., S. W. Leonard, and M. G. Traber. "Vitamin E Kinetics and the Function of Tocopherol Regulatory Proteins." *Nutrition* 17, no. 10 (2001): 799-805.

Bollag, W. "Vitamin a and Retinoids: From Nutrition to Pharmacotherapy in Dermatology and Oncology." *Lancet* 1, no. 8329 (1983): 860-3.

Brigelius-Flohe, R., and M. G. Traber. "Vitamin E: Function and Metabolism." *FASEB J* 13, no. 10 (1999): 1145-55.

Browne, F. J. "Vitamin B1 in Prevention of Pregnancy Toxaemia." *Br Med J* 1, no. 4292 (1943): 445-6.

Burgoon, C. F., Jr., J. H. Graham, F. Urbach, and R. Musgnug. "Effect of Vitamin a on Epithelial Cells of Skin. The Use of Vitamin a in the Treatment of Diseases Characterized by Abnormal Keratinization." *Arch Dermatol* 87, (1963): 63-80.

Burri, B. J., D. D. Bankson, and T. R. Neidlinger. "Use of Free and Transthyretin-Bound Retinol-Binding Protein in Serum as Tests of Vitamin a Status in Humans: Effect of High Creatinine Concentrations in Serum." *Clin Chem* 36, no. 4 (1990): 674-6.

Cabanillas, F. "Vitamin C and Cancer: What Can We Conclude--1,609 Patients and 33 Years Later?" *P R Health Sci J* 29, no. 3 (2010): 215-7.

Carr, A., and B. Frei. "Does Vitamin C Act as a Pro-Oxidant under Physiological Conditions?" *FASEB J* 13, no. 9 (1999): 1007-24.

Carr, F. H., and E. A. Price. "Colour Reactions Attributed to Vitamin A." *Biochem J* 20, no. 3 (1926): 497-501.

Chen, Y. Derguini, F. Buck J. "Vitamin a in Serum Is a Survival Factor for Fibroblasts." *US National Academy of Science* 94, no. 19 (1997): 10205-10208.

Choi, J., S. W. Leonard, K. Kasper, M. McDougall, J. F. Stevens, R. L. Tanguay, and M. G. Traber. "Novel Function of Vitamin E in Regulation of Zebrafish (Danio Rerio) Brain Lysophospholipids Discovered Using Lipidomics." *J Lipid Res* 56, no. 6 (2015): 1182-90.

"Coffee Is Good for You: From Vitamin C and Organic Foods to Low-Carb and Detox Diets, the Truth About Diet and Nutrition Claims." *Library Journal* 137, no. 3 (2012): 120-120.

Detective, Vitamin. "Vitamin Detective." *Booklist* 111, no. 7 (2014): 13-13.

Dzubow, L. M. "Leg Veins and Stretch Marks. Have They Seen the Light?" *Dermatol Surg* 22, no. 4 (1996): 321.

"Earl Mindell's Vitamin Bible (Book)." *Library Journal* 105, no. 6 (1980): 733.

Efremov, VV. "History of the Discovery of Vitamins by N. I. Lunin." *Vopr Pitan* 3, (1982): 68-72.

Eichler, H. G., W. Raffesberg, S. Gasic, A. Korn, and K. Bauer. "Release of Vitamin B12 from Carrier Erythrocytes in Vitro." *Res Exp Med (Berl)* 185, no. 4 (1985): 341-4.

Elalfy, M. S., M. M. Saber, A. A. Adly, E. A. Ismail, M. Tarif, F. Ibrahim, and O. M. Elalfy. "Role of Vitamin C as an Adjuvant Therapy to Different Iron Chelators in Young Beta-Thalassemia Major Patients: Efficacy and Safety in Relation to Tissue Iron Overload." *Eur J Haematol*, (2015).

Elsaie, M. L., L. S. Baumann, and L. T. Elsaaiee. "Striae Distensae (Stretch Marks) and Different Modalities of Therapy: An Update." *Dermatol Surg* 35, no. 4 (2009): 563-73.

Frei, B., and S. Lawson. "Vitamin C and Cancer Revisited." *Proc Natl Acad Sci U S A* 105, no. 32 (2008): 11037-8.

Garrett, J. "[Therapeutic Use of Vitamin B6]." *Port Med* 38, no. 12 (1954): 669-79.

Glossmann, H. "Vitamin D, Uv, and Skin Cancer in the Elderly: To Expose or Not to Expose?" *Gerontology* 57, no. 4 (2011): 350-3.

Greiller, C. L., and A. R. Martineau. "Modulation of the Immune Response to Respiratory Viruses by Vitamin D." *Nutrients* 7, no. 6 (2015): 4240-4270.

Haugen, Leiv, and Terje Bjornson. *Beta Carotene : Dietary Sources, Cancer and Cognition* Nutrition and Diet Research Progress Series. New York: Nova Biomedical Books, 2009.

Jacobs, E. T., and C. J. Mullany. "Vitamin D Deficiency and Inadequacy in a Correctional Population." *Nutrition* 31, no. 5 (2015): 659-63.

Khillan, J. S. "Vitamin a/Retinol and Maintenance of Pluripotency of Stem Cells." *Nutrients* 6, no. 3 (2014): 1209-22.

Knockel, J., I. B. Muller, S. Butzloff, B. Bergmann, R. D. Walter, and C. Wrenger. "The Antioxidative Effect of De Novo Generated Vitamin B6 in Plasmodium Falciparum Validated by Protein Interference." *Biochem J* 443, no. 2 (2012): 397-405.

Kroner, J. C., A. Sommer, and M. Fabri. "Vitamin D Every Day to Keep the Infection Away?" *Nutrients* 7, no. 6 (2015): 4170-4188.

Mahfouz, M. M., S. Q. Zhou, and F. A. Kummerow. "Vitamin B6 Compounds Are Capable of Reducing the Superoxide Radical and Lipid Peroxide Levels Induced by H2o2 in Vascular Endothelial Cells in Culture." *Int J Vitam Nutr Res* 79, no. 4 (2009): 218-29.

Masuda, M., H. Yamamoto, M. Kozai, S. Tanaka, M. Ishiguro, Y. Takei, O. Nakahashi, S. Ikeda, T. Uebanso, Y. Taketani, H. Segawa, K. Miyamoto, and E. Takeda. "Regulation of Renal Sodium-Dependent Phosphate Co-Transporter Genes (Npt2a and Npt2c) by All-Trans-Retinoic Acid and Its Receptors." *Biochem J* 429, no. 3 (2010): 583-92.

McKenna, M. J., B. F. Murray, M. O'Keane, and M. T. Kilbane. "Rising Trend in Vitamin D Status from 1993 to 2013: Dual Concerns for the Future." *Endocr Connect*, (2015).

Mirkazemi, C., G. M. Peterson, P. C. Tenni, and S. L. Jackson. "Vitamin B12 Deficiency in Australian Residential Aged Care Facilities." *J Nutr Health Aging* 16, no. 3 (2012): 277-80.

"Natural Causes: Death, Lies, and Politics in America's Vitamin and
	Herbal Supplement Industry." *Booklist* 103, no. 7 (2006): 9.

Norum, KR, Grav HJ. "Axel Holst and Theodor Frolich—Pioneers in
	the Combat of Scurvy." *Tidsskr Nor Laegeforen* 122, (2002):
	1686-1687.

Pathak, A., and H. A. Godwin. "Vitamin B 12 and Folic Acid Values in
	Premature Infants." *Pediatrics* 50, no. 4 (1972): 584-9.

Pauling, L. "Vitamin C and Common Cold." *JAMA* 216, no. 2 (1971):
	332.

_____. "Vitamin C and Longevity." *Agressologie* 24, no. 7 (1983):
	317-9.

Pauling, L., R. Anderson, S. Banic, T. K. Basu, G. Kallistratos, A.
	Murata, R. Panush, D. Schmahl, and B. V. Siegel. "Workshop
	on Vitamin C in Immunology and Cancer." *Int J Vitam Nutr
	Res Suppl* 23, (1982): 209-19.

Peters, R. A. "The Vitamin B Complex." *Proc Nutr Soc* 4, no. 2 (1946):
	79-81.

Rice, E. G., J. F. Herndon, E. J. Van Loon, and S. M. Greenberg. "Enhancement of Vitamin B12 Absorption of D-Sorbitol as Measured by Maternal and Fetal Tissue Levels in Pregnant Rats." *Am J Physiol* 193, no. 3 (1958): 513-5.

Rocha, H. A., A. C. Silva, L. L. Correia, J. S. Campos, M. M. Machado, A. J. Leite, and A. J. da Cunha. "Effects of Vitamin a Supplementation on Child Morbidity: A Twenty-Year Time Series Analysis in the Northeastern Region of Brazil." *Matern Child Health J*, (2015).

Rodemeister, S., and H. K. Biesalski. "There's Life in the Old Dog Yet: Vitamin C as a Therapeutic Option in Endothelial Dysfunction." *Crit Care* 18, no. 4 (2014): 461.

Rosenfeld, Luis. "Vitamine-Vitamin. The Early Years of Discovery." *Clinical Chemistry* 43, (1997): 680-685.

Sklan D, Shalit I, Lasebnik N, Spirer Z, Weisman Y. "Retinol Transport Proteins and Concentrations in Human Amniotic Fluid, Placenta, and Fetal and Maternal Sera." *British Journal of Nutrition* 54, (1985): 577-583.

Sokmen, B. B., H. Basaraner, and R. Yanardag. "Combined Effects of Treatment with Vitamin C, Vitamin E and Selenium on the Skin of Diabetic Rats." *Hum Exp Toxicol* 32, no. 4 (2013): 379-84.

Sommerburg, Olaf, Werner Siems, and Klaus Kraemer. *Carotenoids and Vitamin a in Translational Medicine* Oxidative Stress and Disease. Boca Raton, FL: CRC Press/Taylor & Francis Group, 2013.

Srivastav, S., S. K. Singh, A. K. Yadav, and S. Srikrishna. "Folic Acid Supplementation Rescues Anomalies Associated with Knockdown of Parkin in Dopaminergic and Serotonergic Neurons in Drosophila Model of Parkinson's Disease." *Biochem Biophys Res Commun* 460, no. 3 (2015): 780-5.

Teplyi, D. L. "[Effect of Vitamin E on Blood-Brain Barrier Permeability]." *Fiziol Zh SSSR Im I M Sechenova* 65, no. 10 (1979): 1506-12.

Traber, M. G. "Mechanisms for the Prevention of Vitamin E Excess." *J Lipid Res* 54, no. 9 (2013): 2295-306.

Traber, M. G., B. Frei, and J. S. Beckman. "Vitamin E Revisited: Do New Data Validate Benefits for Chronic Disease Prevention?" *Curr Opin Lipidol* 19, no. 1 (2008): 30-8.

Traber, M. G., and D. Manor. "Vitamin E." *Adv Nutr* 3, no. 3 (2012): 330-1.

Traxer, O., M. S. Pearle, B. Gattegno, and P. Thibault. "[Vitamin C and Stone Risk. Review of the Literature]." *Prog Urol* 13, no. 6 (2003): 1290-4.

Vaidya, Vishal S., and Joseph V. Bonventre. *Biomarkers : In Medicine, Drug Discovery, and Environmental Health.* Hoboken, N.J.: Wiley, 2010.

"The Vitamin and Mineral Encyclopedia (Book)." *Library Journal* 115, no. 6 (1990): 106-107.

"Vitamin Discoveries and Disasters: History, Science, and Controversies." *Choice: Current Reviews for Academic Libraries* 47, no. 5 (2010): 924-925.

Watanabe, F., Y. Yabuta, T. Bito, and F. Teng. "Vitamin B(1)(2)-Containing Plant Food Sources for Vegetarians." *Nutrients* 6, no. 5 (2014): 1861-73.

Wuerges, J., S. Geremia, and L. Randaccio. "Structural Study on Ligand Specificity of Human Vitamin B12 Transporters." *Biochem J* 403, no. 3 (2007): 431-40.

Yew, M. L. ""Recommended Daily Allowances" for Vitamin C." *Proc Natl Acad Sci U S A* 70, no. 4 (1973): 969-72.

Young, G. L., and D. Jewell. "Creams for Preventing Stretch Marks in Pregnancy." *Cochrane Database Syst Rev*, no. 2 (2000): CD000066.

Zwicker, J. "[Acid Inhibition Leads to Vitamin B12 Deficiency]." *Med Monatsschr Pharm* 37, no. 5 (2014): 190-1.